SO YOU HAVE AN INVISIBLE FRIEND

(See no god, hear no god, speak no god)

By: NANCY PHILLIPS

COPYRIGHT 2016

FIRST EDITION

All rights reserved under International and Pan-American Conventions. No part of this publication may be reproduced, stored in a retrieval system or transmitted in any form by any means, mechanical, photocopying, recording or otherwise, without the permission of the copyright holder.

Printed in the USA

Imprint: Independently published

ISBN: 9781796937329

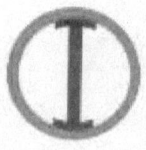

TABLE OF CONTENTS

SO YOU HAVE AN INVISIBLE FRIEND

TABLE OF CONTENTS	iii
PREFACE	vii
INTRODUCTION	xi

    Healing from visual impairment

Chapter 1: VISIBLY INVISIBLE FRIEND — p1

    Sharing my quest
    A good-looking god
    Knock-knock, are you there?

Chapter 2: A FRIEND TO SPEAK TO — p5

    How can I know who is who?
    The making of a good prayer
    The numbers game
    Dissecting a prayer
    The purpose and meaning of prayer
    Science and prayer
    Does God have a plan?
    What have we learned about prayer?

Chapter 3: WHAT CAN I OFFER YOUR FRIEND? — p15

    Does God prefer an offering,
    a sacrifice?
    Abusive behavior
    Are we not heard?
    Proof by lightning

       One way feedback
       Succession of failures

Chapter 4: CAN YOUR FRIEND SPEAK TO ME?   p22

       What have we learned?
       Angels on high
       Moroni, the angel
       Angels and dragons

Chapter 5: YOUR FRIEND'S GREATEST MESSAGE   p29

       Messages called scriptures
       Godly simplifications
       Omniscience and communication
       A litmus test

Chapter 6: SO YOUR FRIEND HAS A BOOK?   p38

       How reliable is your friend's book?
       Who believes in Noah's ark?
       Build a new ark
       The Noachian Paradox
       A layer of humans in the mud
       Consequence for Jesus
       What have we learned?

Chapter 7: THE VALUE OF WRITTEN DOCUMENTS   p45

       If it's written, it's true
       I believe in Nemo and Oz
       Elusive accuracy
       The value of historical texts
       Establishing authentication
       Millions and Billions
       Quoting erroneous texts
       Quoting a non-accredited reference

Chapter 8: EYEWITNESSES THEY SAY   p52

        Gaius Julius Caesar
        Spartacus
        Buddha
        Jesus Christ
        Objective analysis of the Resurrection

Chapter 9: YOUR FRIEND DOES MIRACLES   p62

        What is a miracle?
        Purtill's fantastic criterion
        Benefits from miracles
        Rewards from a biased god
        The simpler the better

Chapter 10: SO WHO KNOWS GOD?   p68

        The '*Knowers*' of god
        Irrelevance
        Why do we need a god?
        Without a god
        Why young adults abandon religion
        The Guilt-forever-syndrome

Chapter 11: DEATH OF THE MINOTAUR   p77

        See no god, hear no god …
        The inaccessible god
        Inaccessism
        Theology, a misnomer
        Life without god

Chapter 12: A TIME FOR HEALING   p87

        Did you say hallucinations?
        Religion and psychotherapy
        Healing abandoned by science

Time wasted to salvation instead of knowledge
Fairytale land

APPENDIX   p98

BIBLIOGRAPHY & SUGGESTED READINGS   p102

Illustration Credits   p104

PREFACE

Early in my search for a publisher, I received an answer to one of my proposals that read, "Thank you but we only accept manuscripts of at least 90,000 words for this category": Well then welcome to the manuscript (and book) that destroys religion in fewer than 40 thousand words.

The purpose of this book is to present to as large a public as possible, the shattering changes in paradigm and the new principle that inevitably appear subsequent to a profound, objective and almost forensic analysis of the claims of institutionalized religion in regards to its god. In consequence, the Philosophy of Religion is abysmally changed. Religion claims to know its god(s). But, in every instance where it should be able to predict where He is or the outcome of a certain event or of a certain prayer, sacrifice, beseeching, healing, etc. it falls short, it fails. Why? So, can religion still convince us that we can see, hear, smell, taste and communicate with its invisible friend?

This is not a long boring theological debate like the thousands already exposed by hundreds of writers. You might wonder why I don't ask religion alone. One of the reasons is that religion has always drowned researchers in quagmires of rhetoric, apologetics and scriptures that often lead nowhere. Religion claims that there is a god and this places the burden of proof on religion; a proof that we are still awaiting after hundreds of years. This is my story of how I learned the arguments and the parries that enabled me to cope with the traps and hurdles that religion has learned to set over the last 3,000 years. But, ironically and by excess, it has developed unwittingly the elements of its own demise.

Confronted by apologists, I would be accused of not being a "scholar", a theologian and therefore incapable of an academic analysis of scriptures. I would concede to this appraisal if I were to engage in yet another interpretation of scriptures such as the thousands that have been attempted by the more scholarly. But this is not what this book is about. After all I am simply applying a form of critical thinking and almost scientific analysis to religion even if it's not without some satire and irony. I much prefer being a satirical skeptic than a "stifled academic who had never risked a thought", to paraphrase James Watson in his *The Double Helix*.

This does not mean that this book is without scholastic merit or without substantiated arguments; it deals a mortal blow to the foundations of religion that, unbeknownst to it, were fragile and fractured from the start. Each of religion's claims is methodically, objectively and relentlessly demolished. Religion is left with no validity, no authenticity and no authority on matters of the divine. It is a revolutionary approach to the analysis of the philosophy of religious doctrine and a condemnation of institutionalized religion as a maleficent, dangerous and pervasive cause and petri dish of millions of neuroses, hallucinations, phobias and other psychological disorders that science neglects purposely because of some sort of taboo. But, with the death of religion there is new hope for healing. Every argument set forth is in response to claims and arguments of truth purported by religious scriptures and Churches. Each argument is set forth with objective, rigorous precision and indisputable accuracy, logic and reason. I have provided a clear and appropriate knowledge exchange strategy for involving all interested parties including potential users of the research within the academic community. I have provided sufficient resource to contribute to a far reaching generational evaluation and debate. All of the data has been properly referenced in an appendix. The few pictures and short iconography is entirely of the author's creation. This book is the result of at least nine years of investigation and research.

There is no deliberate intention of offending anyone despite some irony and mild sarcasm. However, the inevitable conclusions may lead to claims of heresy and even insult to the god of scriptures by fundamentalists of every stripe. There is no reasoning with extremism whatever the subject matter. For obvious similarities, this is the nonfiction equivalent of Dan Brown's, *The Da Vinci Code*. It contains a certain suspense and thrill of the discovery of surprising new paradigms and principles, the consequences of which are disastrous for religion. It reads like a novel whose conclusions are far reaching and transformative. The conclusions arise from a series of objective, rational and sanguine dissections of every claim made by scriptural religion; religion has unknowingly created a god that is so inaccessible that it has unwittingly created the elements of its own destruction. By following the claims of scriptural religion, that it willingly offers, it exposes itself to its own traps. What we discover about Christianity is necessarily true for the other two Judeo-Christian Religions; this is a sweeping paradigm shattering work. Galileo discovered the revolution of the planets about the sun in elliptical orbits thus upsetting the previous religious paradigm by 180 degrees. In this non-fiction book is a paradigm-shattering revolution of ideas that not only flips religious philosophy on its head but decapitates it completely. Prior to Galileo, Copernicus unfortunately wrote in Latin. Consequently, very few people read his work, seeing as few people knew how to read Latin. Galileo understood this and wrote his *Dialogue* in Italian prose and it was an immediate success. I write in English prose and use his dialogue device with the intent of reaching a large audience.

Alas, Science and Philosophy have gotten so bogged down in the petty apologetics and the mires of theological academic tar pits that two thousand years of institutionalized religion have edified, that those who have attempted to see through the complexities deliberately placed as obstacles, have had their vision obscured and impaired to keep them from finding arguments against it. They have lost their way in the maze created for the purpose of confusion. It is easy to get lost in this maze that religion has so well refined.

Dr. Richard Dawkins, as an evolutionary biologist has very eloquently defended the reality of evolution against the arguments of the Creationists. He also defends rationality and logic, but in no way does he even come close to bringing the correct arguments that would wound the institution of religion, as demonstrated by the numerous books he has written and the debates he has participated in to little avail. He has collided with the forbidden walls of religion and only succeeded in getting lost in the maze. Christopher Hitchens criticizes the actions of religion and religious leaders and their influence on modern and historical society. But, he too gets lost in the maze and stops at the forbidden walls, leaving religion relatively unscathed. Dr. Daniel Dennett brings a philosophical and evolutionary approach to the history and the "Phenomenon of religion" but also stops at the forbidden wall of dogmas and claims of religion. Dr. Sam Harris, and Dr. Michael Shermer, battle religion from a neuroscience standpoint, emphasizing rationality and logic: They argue that the existence of moral values, of notions of good and evil are created by the brain and that it does not need religion for that. But, they come up against the forbidden walls as well. They have all come to a brick wall behind which is a formidable maze. They have not seen that religion's walls are sitting on unstable and even fractured substratum. Dr. Bart Ehrman, as a biblical scholar, is the only one who comes close to dismantling the forbidden walls of the institution of religion, but perhaps because he is a believer and involved in the institution itself, he either hesitates or fails to go all the way to the essential conclusion that should appear evident to him. But, at no time have any of them seen that the argument against religion's authority, authenticity or validity, in matters of the divine, is the series of fatal elements unveiled in this quest for freedom from religion

I use the myth of the maze of the ancient Greeks as a metaphor. Following a similar dialogue device as Galileo (1616), the Minotaur represents religion and lies in wait at the center of the maze, ready to pounce on me and destroy my arguments and make of me a believer. But, I follow an Ariadne's thread and manage to penetrate the center of the maze and kill the Minotaur; the thread is a metaphor for a group of anonymous friendly and imaginary religious guides to my quest, to which you are invited.

INTRODUCTION

Life is either a daring adventure, or nothing.
Helen Keller

Hi, my name is Nancy Phillips and this is my story. It all started when I was about 15 and an elderly man came to our home under the guise of sharpening scissors, knives and what not. It turned out that he was a self-appointed missionary who wanted to convert us to his religion. He told us that he had an invisible friend that he could see, hear and converse with. At one point he fell to his knees and began a prayer that I would surmise as "Help these people who are in need of your assistance in seeing you, hearing you and speaking to you".

You see, my father was an atheist and my mother who went to Catholic school, never followed up on the religion. We gave the man some money for his work and sent him off with thankyous for his well wishes. I remember it to this day. I was never really attracted to religion but this incident troubled me. How could a grown man behave as if he could see, hear and speak to an invisible friend? Ever since, I have encountered others. This is when I decided to go on my quest for understanding. After all, I couldn't be the only one that had a visual impairment.

Healing from visual impairment

I have sincerely tried to see their invisible friend but to no avail. I may just need glasses. The most troubling to me though is not that I cannot see Him (or them) but that perfectly respectable persons all around me and around the world can see Him. Most of these people live what we all consider to be normal lives. I have had clerks, cashiers, lawyers, doctors… ask me to come to their homes away from home to meet their invisible friend (sometimes there are more than one friend), so that I can feel content and healed of all my presumed ailments. They call these homes away from home, Churches, Synagogues, Temples, Sacred places and more. I have been to many of them and even those that were out in the woods, on hills, in savannahs, or in deserts. Before I knew that these invisible beings existed, I was perfectly happy and content. However, when I learned that such people as the Pope, the local surgeon, presidents of countries, members of Parliament, of Congress and of armed forces, among others, not only see them/Him but also speak to them and give millions of dollars to others who do also... I started to worry.

It was reassuring when I learned that in the shadows of these powerful and respected 'normal' people are many quiet ones who do not see them either, like me. Once reassured that I was not alone in this visual impairment, I began to question the necessity for some form of healing. None of the answers I have received on this subject has held up to the simplest common-sense analysis. I just need to accept that I am not part of the 'norm'.

Over the years, however, I decided to invite many people who have an invisible friend to help me heal from this horrible deficiency. Many promised to serve as guides to help me navigate the maze of questions I had about all of this. They helped me avoid getting bogged down in the petty apologetics and the mires of theological academic tar pits and created an Ariadne's thread to guide me and without which I would have been devoured by the Minotaur. They were very willing to help and some hoped to see me convert. I told them that they were taking risks with me because, as a scientist for many years, I have become a skeptic and very empirical; I have been visually deficient for too many years. I warned them that I could be very blunt and at times my dissections could be sanguine. But they all acquiesced without hesitation, convinced they could see me heal.

In today's world there is no escaping religion because it is imbedded in every aspect of society and propagates like a virus that we are not yet vaccinated against. I genuinely tried to "see the light" and as a stubborn scientist, I tried to reconcile the dogmas, tenets and explanations given me for why and how I should believe with the rationality I had become accustomed to: But, the natural world has so much logic and the supernatural one has none.

Contrary to what some of you may expect, I did not set out to upset any apple-carts. My quest for truth grew slowly over many years as a sort of leitmotif that spontaneously reoccurred every now and then somewhat like the flue. It's not that it was an unpleasant experience, but it interrupted my other more mundane preoccupations and once it took hold, it would demand my attention and linger on. It would only take an event in the news, a sentence or paragraph in a book, a movie, or just something one might say, to infect my mind and start a fever.

Finally, I decided to go on a quest with the determination of a knight in shining armor to conquer my doubts, fears, deficiencies and demons once and for all. This book is the result of all of these long years of my crusade (for lack of a better word) and of many flue seasons.

Two thousand years of institutionalized religion have so infected science and philosophy that those who have attempted to see through the complexities deliberately placed as obstacles have had their vision obscured and impaired to keep them from finding arguments against it. They have lost their way in the maze created for the purpose of confusion. It is easy to get lost in this maze that religion has so well refined. Navigating the maze successfully is our goal in this quest you are invited to. Ariadne's thread is almost invisible to the person that has been blinded by religious superfluities and smoke screens. But once you find the thread, it assuredly leads you to the inner sanctum, a change of paradigm, a new principle as well as to the true and inevitable death of religion.

The results surprised even me because in my wildest dreams I never thought I would discover so much of what was right under my (runny) nose all along. I invite you to follow in my footsteps and experience for yourself the astonishment at the discovery of the inevitable and shattering conclusions resulting from this journey. So come along on a quest I began several decades ago. You will understand that those most in need of healing are not those you may expect.

CHAPTER 1

VISIBLY INVISIBLE FRIEND

Sharing my quest

My first question to the "normal" people who have an invisible friend is, "What is your friend's name?" The answers I get vary quite a bit but most often they agree on one name and that is "God", a generic name to which too many refer to as if it were a foregone conclusion that it is their god and no one else's. However, depending on who I speak to, I find myself confronted with Allah, Yahweh, Jehovah, Elohim, Jesus, Manitou, Wakan Tanka, Vishnu, Kali, and many more. Unanimously, they all agree that this god (take your pick) is their friend and he wants them to believe in him, worship him, and pray to him.

I look about me and I notice that millions of human beings around the world see an invisible friend. But oddly enough they do not believe the same things, they do not wear the same clothes, pray like others pray, worship like others worship and what is more, they have a different friend than others do. How can I explain this? I am told over and over again that there is only one. This troubles me. I find this one question particularly unavoidable; how can I explain that different people see different invisible friends? So, what is the answer? Those afflicted with visual impairment are definitely not the ones I expected.

Because the people to whom I have spoken the most were Christian, I will focus on the Bible to shorten the length of this book. Therefore the God mentioned most often in this book, unless otherwise specified, is the Judeo-Christian-Islamic one since this is the god of the main scriptural religions of the world. In fact, technically speaking the god of Judaism, of Christianity, and of Islam is one and the same despite different aliases. What is more, He is responsible for dictating and/or inspiring the Torah, the Bible and the Qur'an, the very foundations of each religion. What we will learn about one of these religions will necessarily apply to the other two.

A good-looking god

In most temples and churches of scriptural religions, old and new, there is a special place, a special room, equivalent to the so-called *holy of holies*. Whether reserved to the high priest or not, it is where god is sensed resting and present. In the temple of Jerusalem, it was a room barred by a huge curtain and lit by a small window in the ceiling, as well as candles, and where incense burned. As seen from a skeptic's point of view, it is fair to ask if god is present there and at what time of the day or week. In any given room of a church, temple, synagogue, mosque, etc., just how does one know when god is there? This is a fair question to ask a priest, pastor, or rabbi, etc., when invited to penetrate the *lieu* of cult.

Just what does God look like, how could we identify Him if He were present? Religious scriptures and oral traditions are full of long lists of attributes (powers, characteristics, qualities) of a specific god. I will not take time to analyze the plethora of attributes listed in most scriptural religions but only focus on those that are the most prominent and that inevitably contradict each other. So, let's take a quick short look at the scriptures. They offer us a list of God's attributes. The first attribute that concerns us is that He is **invisible (Genesis 32:22-30; Exodus 24:9-11; 1 Timothy 1:17; Deuteronomy 4:15; Job 9:11; Matthew 6:6; Romans 1:20; Colossians 1:15; Hebrews; 11:27; 1 John 4:12).**

It should not surprise anyone therefore, that when the special chamber or room was finally accessible to the public especially after abandonment or destruction of the edifice or the religion, it was… empty. Even today the same principle applies and one can assuredly say that the god of scriptural religions is still but an empty chamber. It appears (no pun intended) that this god is obviously invisible. After all and to be fair, religion does tell us that the Bible says,

- He is **immaterial (John 4:23-24)**
- He is **undetectable (Job 11:7-8 & 26:14 & 37:23; Psalms 145:3; Isaiah 40:28; 55:8-9; 1 Timothy 6:16)**

Religion claims to know its god(s). But, we will see that in every instance where it should be able to predict where He is or the outcome of a certain event or of a certain prayer, sacrifice, beseeching, healing, etc. it falls short, it fails. Why? So, can religion still convince me and help me see this invisible friend? For the time being He is visibly invisible.

You must already be dreading and expecting a long boring theological debate like the millions already exposed by hundreds of writers. I want to put your fears to rest. You might wonder why I don't ask religion alone. One of the reasons is that religion has always drowned researchers in quagmires of rhetoric, apologetics and scriptures that often lead nowhere. Religion claims that there is a god, this places the burden of proof on religion and we will be faced with what religion has to say about Him sooner or later as we progress. Where does one start analyzing religion and what does one analyze?

"I hear you my friend! Stay calm! I seem to be empirically brushing aside with a quick sweep of the hand the entire scriptures and declaring them of no interest. It is common to admit that the scriptures are true from the get-go. But the premise here is that they are false, or questionable, until proven true or worthy of authority. This is the essential premise of this book. We will obviously come to an analysis of the key points related to scriptures in due time. This is just a different approach and the basis for a change of paradigm."

Knock-knock, are you there?

As an archeologist I have visited a great many holy sites such as Lascaux (the real one), Stonehenge, Olduvai Gorge, the Medicine Wheel site in Wyoming, The Black Hills of the Dakotas, a small chapel in an extinct volcanic crater, numerous cathedrals in Europe, etc. I have seen believers call their invisible friend by name or ring a bell, burn incense, play a drum, a flute, sing, psalmody, and much more. But, even here, the question still lingers; how do we know this invisible friend is there when we beckon him? It has always astonished me to hear religion and religious people ask me to believe in their dogmas or scriptures which clearly state that this god is invisible and yet they expect me to see him. They say that I need to be in the spirit or that the spirit must be in me... which makes no sense to me but plenty to them. We have a ways to go.

The epitome is when a religious person argues that a blind scientist would be unable to do any research or true science. But, Science can discover without seeing whereas religion seems to be able to "see" without ever discovering. Scientists have observed microscopic reality without ever having seen it per se. No one has ever seen an atom or even a molecule *de visu* but science has recorded their reactions, their trajectories, their electrical charges and it can predict their behavior every time an atom or a molecule are placed in the presence of other known substances; Chemistry and Physics work together. One last example is how astrophysicists can know what the mineral composition of a moon or planet is through the analysis of the light that comes from it without ever having to set foot on it. It is this predictability through distinct technical processes and methods which gives Science its phenomenal advantage over religion in matters of detecting and understanding the realities of the world.

As it is suggested by authors such as Victor Stenger [1], Daniel Dennett [2] and others, perhaps the unique god hypothesis is a failed one. In their view it is a failed hypothesis in the light of the laws of Physics and Nature in general. But they consider the god of Physics and not the god described by religion and by these "normal" people who say that they can see him. These visually acute people are the ones that I want to have explain to me just who this invisible friend of theirs is. Are they endowed with supernatural powers? After all, let us not forget that science deals with natural phenomena and religion with supernatural phenomena.

Alas, I have to accept the fact that I may never be able to see Him since their god is not visible, not material and undetectable. I am all the more intrigued by the questions, "How do they know He is there, how do they communicate with Him and know what He wants"? So, for the time being, I will focus on how to communicate with Him. Religion claims to know its god and I am willing learn if it is willing to teach. Are you willing to test your faith, discover new ways of perceiving a truth, or even the truth, or of simply not being visually impaired about religion? Then keep following Ariadne's thread with me as our quest evolves. This is just the beginning of our quest.

CHAPTER 2

A FRIEND TO SPEAK TO

How can I know who is who?

Religion and the people who say that they see their invisible friend (god) have trouble showing Him to me. I feel better already about my own visual impairment. Despite this dilemma, religion will invariably tell me that it can and has communicated with its god. The aspects of this communication will be our greatest inquiry.

Religion and religious people with extrasensory visual acuity tell me that despite my visual impairment I can communicate with him as they do through prayer. So, my next question is, "to which of these invisible friends do I pray to?" In other words, "how can I know which one is the right invisible friend (god) and which is the right religion?"

So, I ask my religious guide, "How can you be sure that your interpretation, your practice, and your denomination, is sufficiently informed and correct to be able to save your soul? By trying to guess at who the real god is and what this god wants are you not exposing yourself to the risk of mortal errors?" This is where my guide offers a solution that consists of asking god himself to give me a sign. "Only He can tell you which religion and which denomination has the truth", says my guide. That is an interesting point. Unfortunately, awaiting an answer, a sign, can take forever. Besides, what about all of those other people out there who have asked this question and who have received different signs for the same question? It is easy to conclude that this solution is illusory and even disingenuous, in all due respect. Why? Because it means that God would give the same answer to all who would ask this question. If this were the case, God would have surely straightened things out by now and there would be only one true religion on the face of the Earth, after all "God may be mysterious, said Einstein, but he is certainly not mischievous".

My religious guide insists! "Oh, all right, I will play along with this prayer stuff because I am open-minded and fair-play. But, I will not pray to any of these invisible friends myself because I don't want to put any of them on the spot", I say. It's not surprising that even today people from all walks of life declare that not only do they see god but God speaks to them and that we, in turn, can speak to God; then let's start by asking these people just how God speaks (or spoke) to us or them, and how we can respond? They say it is through prayer, offerings and sacrifice; surely these have been a way to communicate with God? But let us agree that simply hearing voices that no one else can hear or record is not a valid argument. On top of my first dilemma (I can't see these friends) it's surprising that I can't hear them either. Decidedly, I seem to have a second infirmity; a hearing deficit.

The making of a good prayer

Just what does God have to say about this? According to Christianity's scriptures, to which we must refer for the sake of our inquiry, we find a few answers given directly through the presumed words of Jesus. In Matthew chapter 6, he says "Pray in secret, don't go to the synagogue, pray in your closet (in your home discretely), shut the door (don't show off) and pray to your Father in secret for He sees you (in secret). Do not use vain repetitions; God can hear you, once is enough. Do not forget that your Father knows what things you have need of before you ask him for them." Ironically this last sentence almost nullifies the need for prayer altogether since if you needed it and haven't gotten it, whatever it is you need, wouldn't you have received it without praying if you deserved it?

Please notice the inconsistency and contradiction in this alleged statement by Jesus. The scriptures say that God does not seem to appreciate and listen to those who make fanfare of their faith when they pray. He would rather that you pray in your home, discretely, but he is flattered that you build churches, temples, Mosques and synagogues, and gather to pray regularly. It could be that the priests need a place to stay and gather your donations? We have here a god who knows what you need, but who does not give it to you, at least when you think you need it. The answer of course is that he knows better than you do what you should have which means that you shouldn't even ask. However he likes to hear you ask and see you bow down to him.

I have to admit that there are good clinical indications that show that prayer as well as meditation and other therapeutics have very potent psychological healing potential. What counts is that prayer, like meditation, helps an ailing person become aware and conscious of their condition and seems to stimulate numerous functions in the body that tend to help it to recover by sometimes regulating the immune system. It can alleviate anxieties, stress, and it can modify behavior, eating habits, and other factors that may have led to the condition in the first place. Prayer can be a very good practice if identified with harmonization of one's health, spirit, or so-called soul or some transcendent part of one's being if one believes in such things.

However, just what evidence is there for the efficacy of prayer? Ironically, I have often watched people engage in prayer by lowering their heads, putting their hands together, closing tightly their eyes, holding their hands in the air, holding other person's hands, standing, sitting, dancing, jumping to music, playing instruments, smoking tobacco, and many more behaviors. Which of these works the best and pleases this god the most? Is there one type of prayer that really works? Could it just be the amount of praying and not so much the style?

The Apostle Paul is suspected to have said, "We know that God does not answer prayers of sinners". But, since from the very start (Adam & Eve) we are all sinners, this could explain why no one seems to get answers to their prayers, at least when they think they deserve them; any answers that have the appearance of being results of prayers are maybe just that, "appearances".

What then is a good prayer? What are the criteria, the characteristics of a good prayer? What are the consequences or results that one may expect from a good prayer?

The numbers game

When people think of a prayer that will have some weight and can set off a response they often think in terms of numbers. As a skeptic even I would have this instinctive gut feeling that a gathering of people would have more weight in getting what we want from God than if we prayed individually. So then, our first criteria would be sheer numbers. The more we are the merrier, or should I say the better the odds of getting God to do something special. The internet fizzles with Facebook postings asking people for prayers and an Amen. Does this really work and is it ethical? Does it fall under the edicts of a religion? Does grouping together our lottery tickets, make our odds of winning any better? Does gathering in large numbers in a church, a synagogue, a temple, a battle field, a street, make our odds of getting a miracle any better? The sheer number of historical examples demonstrates that this is an illusion. There are literally millions of examples of which I will give at least one well documented one.

Tens of thousands of people prayed across all America to save the life of Teri Schiavo who was in a vegetative state for years in Florida, USA, but she died (March 31, 2005) [3]; this is a sad but perfect illustration. Bad things happen to good people and praying is of no avail no matter how many prayers. Prayer appears to be an illusion and merely the expression of our dysfunctional mysticism and irrationality. But, to be more objective let us examine methodically some key examples.

Dissecting a prayer

I heard a man interviewed on a prayer program and he was asked to tell the story of how he and his wife survived a tornado, somewhere in the USA, whereas four of his less fortunate neighbors died. This sincerely thankful individual said that the storm came while he and his wife were asleep, tore the roof off their house and turned their bed upside down. He explained that the mattress and box spring probably saved their lives by protecting them from flying debris. He said something to the order of: "I could feel the mattress and box spring upon us and though I tried to stand up in the midst of the storm a force held me down. It was as though the hand of God was protecting us by keeping us covered and out of harm's way". Of course these are not his exact words but the general meaning is there. He went on to say that surely God had saved them. After all, during this horrifying event, he had kept on praying. "So, you see, God does answer prayer." Even the host of the show warmly agreed. It never occurred to either one of them that some simple explanations may have been the answer to some of the sequences of events. It never occurred to them that a good King or Queen-sized bed weighs enough to hold anybody down especially when the wind is blowing over it at over 100 miles an hour. No wonder he felt something holding him down.

As for the rest of his mysticism, he overtly suggests that god saved his life. Then why did He not save the lives of the four other people? Could it be that the others were not praying enough or with enough fervor, that they were not saying the right prayer or that they were not praying to the same and the right god? Could it be that they were not good Christians, were they sinners, did they not go to church that Sunday…? Does this man really think that he is worthier to live than the four others who died? One is left with these horrible questions as to why God, the all-powerful, the all merciful did not save anyone else but them. These people obviously have no shame. If some poor member of the devastated families, relatives to those who died, had heard this broadcast, what would his/her reaction have been? Moreover, if god is as powerful as these perfect people like to repeat, then why did he not just simply, either stop the storm all together, or at least force it into some other direction that would have avoided killing these people or anybody else for that matter? Surely, these worthier people have an interpretation for even this.

This is just but one example among thousands. But this man speaks as a witness and for that reason he must act as one before the law. His testimony of the storm is in itself substantiated, but as to the intervention of God it would never hold up before any judge or jury; it is not provable, it is subjective, circumstantial and rests on his interpretations, his convictions alone. It is to say the least disingenuous to me that he intertwines his interpretations with the physical, natural storm event. This is a perfect example of why it is necessary to demand objective, judicially admissible evidence for these types of so-called witnessing where people subversively introduce their religious interpretations into perfectly natural events.

The purpose and meaning of prayer

The previous example is but one of many where the purpose of the prayer is obviously to get this god to save our skin. On the radio and on TV (in some countries at least) you can hear people praying for those who call in their prayer requests. How touching it is then to hear the host say, "… and we pray for John who has cancer, and for Ruth and Bob who need funds, and for Catherine who is trying to stop drinking and …" This list goes on without end. In sports, quite often players repeatedly acknowledge that god was on their side, and of course not on the side of the others, by saying something to the order of "we prayed and prayed, God gave us the strength, victory and God did this, and God gave us that". Is this the meaning of prayer? Is this the goal of praying? Does one pray to obtain some sort of favor, some sort of gift or present from god? Is god some sort of Santa Claus? Therefore, by being good and faithful, and prayerful, we may hope to get what we wished (sorry; prayed for). But, why would God who is supposed to be fair and just, take sides in a battle or even a game? Could he be biased?

A medical doctor presented an account of how he drowned in a boating accident, went to heaven and was brought back to life by a godly intervention after onlookers pulled him from the waters and gave him CPR. He wrote a book on his experiential accident in which he went to and returned from heaven (or what he perceived as heaven). We can wonder if he would have regained consciousness if no one had been there to give him CPR. Secondly, if he had regained consciousness alone, would this still have been some sort of miracle, or just a happenstance? This is not something science can experiment with; there is no way of verifying. But, this is something a doctor, who is a scientist, should have considered. There is no excuse for a medical doctor with a scientific background to give unbridled liberty to his or her religious hallucinations without some attempt at a short critical and objective analysis. It is an abomination for a doctor to pretend that divine healings, dispensed by an all loving, all-merciful, all-powerful deity, exist. Why then would one be a doctor in the first place if such a deity exists? A wounded accident or war victim should recover with a simple prayer. Such a victim should receive a simple miracle at any and all times. I would cringe at the thought of doctors who would tell their patients, "never fear, if you die, god will make everything OK, you won't feel a thing and heaven is a wonderful place that awaits you". In other words, "I will do all I can to save you, but if I can't, it's no big deal".

The blatant arrogance of some people enables them to pretend that they have been the worthy recipients of heavenly favors that saved their lives while other people less fortunate (or should we say, less worthy?) died. The reality of historical events shows and proves that millions of poor victims, innocent or not, should have survived through divine healing the horrors of wars and accidents but did not despite many prayers. Religion is a school where self-righteousness and arrogance run amuck. It is the right of anyone to have certain beliefs and a certain faith. However, without due process of evidence, it is outrageous to want to impose an illusion such as healing prayer and favoritism-prayer upon the rest of us who may have other worldviews. It is so simple to keep it to yourself and only express it inside the privileged religious communities that teach, covet and incubate these insidious ideas. There is neither need, nor excuse for all the types of demonstrations, provocations and rebellions against simple common-sense laws that discourage or prohibit religious prayers in public schools or even on the athletic field.

Surely there are some people more worthy and righteous than others. Oh, but surely there are good causes to fight and go to war over. Surely it is righteous to go to war to force people to understand that slavery is an inhuman endeavor. But, how can a religion not condemn slavery let alone a war, a fratricide, when it knows that killing is a sin (the sixth commandment)? Why is there no commandment that prohibits slavery? In the days of this legendary Moses, slavery was already widely practiced. One would think that an omniscient, omnipotent and all-merciful god would dictate a commandment against such a horrible thing. All of this has been said over and over but, why does this not trouble religion or the religious at large? The people who fought in the American civil war had faith in the same god, in the same scriptures. How is it that an all-mighty, all-merciful, all-loving god would intervene to help a team or an individual win a game and not intervene to save the lives of millions of wounded soldiers despite incalculable healing prayers? How is it that this same god would not be able to open a few concentration camp doors to free its prisoners? We still have more questions than answers.

Science and prayer

Does Science have anything to say in the matter? What could Science possibly have to say, this is a matter of faith?
Well Science has already said quite a bit about it. As early as August 1, 1872 to be exact, Sir Francis Galton, a British Scientist pronounced an eloquent analysis of prayer and presented a statistical study that demonstrated the inefficacy of prayer. He demonstrates the vanity of the idea that pious prayer can offer special providences (interferences of god) to those who pray in the name of a particular god and in the case of Christians, to Jesus. He concludes that prayer can only be universal or god would be biased and respond to only some people and not all. Therefore, the corollary, the universality of prayer, either proves too much or it destroys religion. Indeed, one is then compelled to admit that the prayers of Pagans, Heathens, and the rest of the world are answered in the same way as those who follow religious orthodox rituals, in which case why bother with religion. I encourage you to research and read more on the clairvoyance and scientific prudence in his studies.

If this is not enough, a more recent three-year Study of the Therapeutic Effects of Intercessory Prayer (STEP) [4], was published in April of 2006 is the largest scientific application to the study of the influence of prayer on the wellbeing of 1,800 patients undergoing heart-bypass surgery. The study was paid by the John Templeton Foundation and cost $2.4 million. The research team included doctors and clergy from six institutions including Harvard Medical School and the Mayo Clinic in the USA.

The team found no differences in survival or complication rates in the groups being prayed for than compared with those who did not receive prayers. They even found a 7% higher rate of complications in one subgroup of patients who were prayed for and knew it, whereas all other groups were not informed that someone was praying for them.

Does God have a plan?

Could all of what we have just analyzed and discovered be explained because God has a plan? Let me give you two examples, among thousands.

The first example took place in Seminole Heights, Florida in July, 2012 [5]. United Methodist Church Pastor Sharon Davis' nightly walk is a routine she is well known for. At the end, she sits in the same spot outside Seminole Heights to pray for the community and the church and to reflect on everything she has been working on. But on a Sunday night, her walk ended with a surprise from above.

Pastor Sharon Davis sustained serious injuries after a tree limb fell on her as she prayed. One might wonder what she was praying for and why God was not on guard. As Davis prayed, she heard a cracking sound coming from overhead. Before she could even look up, church members said, she was struck by a falling tree limb on the church's steps. She doesn't remember being struck, but she remembers waking up on the ground, according to church member Beni Blankenship. "The tree limb threw her back and down, breaking her clavicle in three places and cutting her head open pretty badly," Blankenship said. "Other than that she was just really sore but doing OK."

The large tree limb is believed to have been weakened by the wrath of Tropical Storm Debby which hit the city of Tampa. Luckily for Davis, there happened to be a neighbor outside their home who saw the event unfold and was able to dial 911 within minutes. Davis was hospitalized and ironically just asked for prayers for healing. Obviously, the first prayers (hers) were either not worded correctly or did not include a clause of protection from falling branches.

Secondly, in April of 2001 a missionary in Peru, his wife and 4-year-old daughter were flying to a remote mission [5]. Their plane was taken for a drug cartel delivery of drugs. The Peruvian air force shot at the plan to for it to land. The missionary's wife and daughter were killed by the same bullet. They briefly prayed before being shot down and God must have certainly been looking after them, after all they were Christian missionaries. Later, reflecting on the tragedy at the funeral of his wife and daughter, the husband said that God had made other plans for them and his relief came from the thought that his wife and daughter were now with the Lord (their god). Therefore, "God has a plan for all of us and He loves us all" was what this man insinuated as a conclusion. Unfortunately, if this proclamation that God has a plan is true then free will is an illusion. Moreover, you can pray until you are blue in the face, but if God has a plan for you to die, then it is of no avail to pray. This man's conclusion conveniently absolves him from responsibility.

One of my religious guides explained to me that there is free will despite God's plan conundrum if one considers the possibility of a multiverse or multi-universes. You would still be able to choose and the consequences of your choice would play out in one of the multiverses. However, this would mean that this god would have an infinite number of plans and not just one. This would also mean that He would not have to worry about what might happen to you now that He has covered all of His bases: surely somewhere, one of His plans fits the bill. This would still be a devastating blow to the utility of prayer because the odds of your being, at the moment of your prayer (6), in just the right universe to receive a response and/or a healing would be as good as zero. What is more, the Bible does not speak of anything remotely akin to a multiverse; this is at best a modern science conjecture/hypothesis. Furthermore, the scriptures speak of one plan, not of an infinite number of them.

What have we learned about prayer?

A careful analysis of presumed answers to prayers shows that those who are the recipients of these answers are as random a group as one that would have been chosen by pulling names out of a hat. Decidedly, the number of people praying and the number of prayers is of no influence. Therefore, prayer alone cannot (as yet) be identified with a means of direct or indirect communication with god. Until the day that substantiated, unequivocal evidence of communication with God through prayer is found, not only can no one claim to have communicated with God through prayer but no one or no religion can claim the exclusivity of any access to God in this manner.

If these statistics were not enough, what dysfunctional god would on the same day, after profuse prayers, save the life of a pet cat and allow a young child to die of an abominable disease and in agonizing pain? In what kind of horrifying 'plan' does this statistic fit? Therefore, those who stubbornly refuse to admit this reality and continue to have faith in the illusion of prayer should keep it to themselves and not be allowed to present it as a viable means of communication with God.

By the way, is god not doing his job or what? Why must someone always remind him, through prayer, of what he has to do? These prayerful people say, 'God is all-powerful, he has plans for you and me, he rewards the righteous and punishes evil (the Santa Claus syndrome)' and yet he seems to forget (or might forget) little Billy or Ruth and Bob or Ann or John or even the neighbor's cat if we don't pray constantly for them. So, should we look into impeaching this god and maybe finding another one who would not need all of these constant reminders and who would finally do what some claim he can do?

But, perhaps there are other means of communication?

I do not believe in prayer the way institutionalized religions present it but I find this one particularly suited for the conclusion of this chapter: It is philosophically very beautiful and contains much of the substance of this book. It is a quote from the work of John Michael Crichton (1942 – 2008):

For all we ought to have thought and have not thought,

>All we ought to have said and have not said,

>All we ought to have done and have not done,

>I pray thee god for forgiveness.

CHAPTER 3

WHAT CAN I OFFER YOUR FRIEND?

Does God prefer an offering, a sacrifice?

We have just seen that prayer is not a proven means of communication with God. It is too aleatory. There is no admissible evidence that God answers prayers. But, some people continue to think that by adding a sacrifice or offering to a prayer, ever so small, they will obtain the blessing of God; the car, the money, the girl/boy, the power and so forth. Here again God and the Church are the ultimate ATM's of happiness. By the way, I have not yet healed from neither of my two impairments.

So, what can one offer god? In Matthew Chapter 6 of the Christian scriptures, God likes to see us fast, even if he gives us sustenance (bread) every day. Moreover, we should not be hypocrites about it and go about sad and looking hungry to show off the fact that we are fasting. On the contrary, let us be discrete about this; just go about town "with oil on your head and a clean face". Others instead of fasting have offered portions of their own flesh in the past and some still do today. Some offer an animal or even several. Some offer blood, guts, heads, feathers, and whole paraphernalia of animal remains. These offerings are either buried, or burned and sometimes worn and so forth. Some fervent believers have even sacrificed their own kin. "Human sacrifice is the epitome of the inevitable escalation of the concept of communitarian sacrifice", an anonymous author wrote.

One of Hollywood's all-time classics is "King Kong". In this story a young virgin is given in sacrifice to Kong, the giant gorilla, in the hopes that Kong will spare the rest of the village. In another film, Chieftains cut open men's chests to extract their hearts so that a god will bring rain and spare the tribe from famine. The examples of sacrifices, whether mythical or historically true, abound. Surely sacrificing a virgin to Kong is not quite moral, but if it saves the rest of the tribe it is a necessity. Moreover, if the virgin, after some coaxing, accepts, it falls under altruism, no? Surely sacrificing a virgin to an active volcano, suspected to be a god, an intelligent (though sometimes cruel) entity, is moral and useful. Surely sacrificing men, women and children to a deity, a higher entity, is moral and useful. After all, better them than me or the rest of the tribe, right? Countless consenting individuals have sacrificed themselves for altruistic, patriotic, religious, political reasons and more. Some of these reasons can be seen as morally praiseworthy, others not. When is sacrifice philosophically and morally wrong? When is sacrifice just plain stupid?

This brings up the particular question of the possibility of any individual, and the religion as a whole, to communicate with this entity or entities. Whether this entity is called "King Kong", Krakatau, Marduc, Thor, Pele, Zeus, Poseidon, Quetzalcoatl or any of the other countless entities of human history, how does one communicate and know if the communication works? One simple way is if the sacrifice(s) brings the expected result such as rain, the end of an eruption or the dissipation of an eminent threat. Then sacrifice could be considered as inevitable (though abominable) collateral damage. It is of course usually a last recourse after prayers have been exhausted in many cases. But, inevitably prayer and sacrifice have the same limitations and absurd logic.

Abusive behavior

Religion turns right around to say, "It is not so much how you pray, when you pray, where you pray, what is important is who you pray or sacrifice to. Though if you do not come to church next Sunday you'll go to hell; or if you do not go to mosque this week, we'll dress a fatwa against you and have you sacredly killed"; please note that in this latter example, God never does the killing or punishing, it's always a henchman.

In the Bible, one of the patriarchs (Abraham) is about to sacrifice his own son to prove to God his allegiance (Genesis 22:1-2). What manner of man would deliberately sacrifice one of his own children simply to show his allegiance to a god who can (we are told) see for himself the conduct of this man and know his heart is sincere, if indeed it is? What kind of irrationality is this? In addition, why would any decent person or religion offer this behavior as an example to follow? This type of behavior is as despicable as that of any father who abuses his children and as punishable by human secular laws which have been created recently, in terms of our human history, by secular entities more interested in earthly justice than in heavenly irrationalities. How can we find a god who abuses his son by lethal sacrifice, worthy of worship and moral authority?

Most religions acknowledge that this entity (or principal) has everything in its power, possesses everything; in which case it is not necessary to offer god what is already his. Therefore, it is useless and senseless to offer it anything substantial, besides you cannot out-give God, like religion ironically likes to repeat. Sacrifice and more importantly, human sacrifice, is not only dysfunctional abusive behavior but it should shock our deepest moral fiber. One can argue that sacrifice and prayer are not absurd nor wrong nor cruel if they respond to the requirements of a deity. However, what benevolent all loving god would set prerequisites to his all merciful and all loving care or refuse his aid or even hold back his protection and healing until certain hurdles are jumped, or certain conditions are met? Logically none!

Are we not heard?

On the basis of God's attributes, hang on to your seat.

If God is omnipotent there is nothing He cannot do. If he is omniscient He knows the past the future and the present: He knows what we want, what we need, and if we are suffering. If He is omnibenevolent He can relieve suffering wherever it occurs. But God cannot possess certain attributes all at the same time because they are mutually exclusive. How can that be, might you ask?

Philosophers have demonstrated that if God is omniscient, He cannot be simultaneously omnipotent. If the New York Twin Towers were inscribed to collapse in the future, there is nothing God could do about it. Either God cannot see the future (not omniscient) but can change it (Omnipotent) as it happens, or He can see the future (Omniscient) but then cannot change it (not omnipotent).

If God is omniscient He knows when people are suffering, how they are suffering, and how that suffering may be healed. Obviously, if He does not know of the suffering, he cannot be omniscient.

If He is omnipotent, He is capable of any intervention even if He is busy with something godly important. He should be able to postpone or void the business at hand, and act without regard to it, to heal the person in need. However, if He is not omniscient also, He may not know who needs help which may explain why everyone is not healed. If He is omnibenevolent, He is devoted to relieving the pain of all of those who suffer. But for this He needs to know who is suffering.

Our experience of life shows us that He does not relieve everyone whether they pray for it or not. Why then does He not simply relieve all who suffer? Could it be that He makes the choice to relieve only those who pray? This is inconceivable since He is all-merciful. But, He does not even heal all those who pray either because He may not know who is praying. This tends to prove that despite the fact that He can potentially be omnipotent and omnibenevolent, He is either not simultaneously omniscient (doesn't know who suffers and prays) or He does not hear prayers at all. But then, if He does not hear prayers, He is not omnipotent. Quite the quagmire!

This can only mean that God cannot possess certain attributes at the same time. So, which of these three attributes does God have? Why does religion not know this and why does it insist that He has all three? The answer is that scriptures are errant in this matter. What is more, this indicates that religion does not know its God. But, for the matter at hand, it also means that God does not hear our prayers, does not heed our sacrifices or He is incapable of fulfilling them. It could well be that we simply, for some yet unknown reason, cannot communicate with Him. In any case the results are the same; in other words, if we don't get the answer we should expect from this god for our prayers and sacrifice, it is as if we never prayed at all. This proves that prayer and sacrifice are basically useless.

Have you heard about the National Day of Prayer established quite some time ago in the USA? It calls on all people of different faiths in the United States to pray in their own way for the nation and its leaders. It is held on the first Thursday of May each year. It is not a public holiday. In recent years, more than 30,000 prayer gatherings are conducted by about 40,000 volunteers across the United States. Two million people are presumed to participate in this call to prayer. It includes such themes as, "For your Great Name's Sake! Hear us...Forgive us...Heal us!" If you remember my statement in the introduction of this book, I felt no need for healing from the start. Just what do we need healing from? It appears that this day of prayer is another attempt by religion at perpetuating the paranoia of the Guilt-forever-syndrome or the Repentance-forever-syndrome that we will examine later (see Chapter 8). Whatever our "sins" and "errors", surely this gathering of millions could be more usefully used to obtain some form of reassurance that our prayers are getting through.

How difficult would it be to have people pray for a sign from God? After all this is what my religious guides told me to do. An unequivocal sign such as stopping all machines for about a half hour like in the movie

The Day the Earth Stood Still (1951) by Harry Gilmore. Or how about asking Him to cure all of the patients of cancer in a given Hospital, city or country at a given time? The possibilities are endless. Surely, with all of these people praying at once and of all faiths, we should certainly obtain a distinct positive and unequivocal response. If such a massive prayer should not succeed, then perhaps the healing we need is of illusions and delusions of an all-powerful and all-loving God or, at least, of one that hears our prayers. But, religion says that faith is to precede the miracle and miracles are not to precede the faith yet when it tries to authenticate the divinity of Jesus it resorts quickly to his miracles including the resurrection. This is not a tempting of God, but simply a test of efficacy of prayer. But, of course, if individual prayer is not efficacious then how can it be in large numbers? I see some of my guides shrugging their shoulders and saying that this is just a word game and that "theology" is much more than this.

Proof by lightning

Do you want to prove that prayer is a real and functional means of communication with God and that this god is all powerful or omnipotent? I have a simple solution. Arrange for all religious people of all religions and denominations to pray all at the same time for a week, with offerings, sacrifices and anything they usually do. Ask them to pray god that He send us but one small, short, precise and unequivocal E-mail, in English, telling us that there is only one religion, telling us what that religion is. Moreover, they could also ask god to stop sending henchmen to do the dirty work for him (ex. Charlie Hebdo). On the contrary, ask him to send a simple E-mail to those who deserve his wrath that reads, "You will be struck by lightning next Monday at 10 am", signed God. After which the condemned does get struck that day and that hour. Now if that does not prove that prayer works, that god is almighty and if it does not convert everybody to religion, I'll eat my hat.

The bottom line here is, are we any closer today to knowing what an entity wants? Are we in any better situation to access a god, any gods? It appears clear that rituals including prayer and sacrifice do not allow for effective communication between Man and God.

One-way Feedback

If indeed sacrifice, prayer and other tenets of religions have no more validity or unequivocal substance than what we have exposed, it is not only arrogant to think (and claim) that one has a direct 'phone-line' to God through prayer but it is also a dangerous game, giving people false hope. When people's prayers seemingly go unanswered, it is an insult to them, to their families and even to God to say "it simply did not fit God's plan". This means, "it's going to happen whether you pray or not". This is in complete contradiction with the idea of praying in the first place.

Prayer and sacrifice have no meaning nor purpose if there is no rational feedback. We are fools to think that if we win a game, get the car we dreamed of, succeed in our profession or any other worldly event, that God has anything to do with it unless God takes sides; how could He if He is just and fair? Moreover, we have no right to profess this unless there is a rational and indisputable accessibility to God and vice versa.

This is where most of our religious problems started thousands of years ago. When a man deliberately or inadvertently duped people into thinking he could converse with god(s), the tribe elevated this man to social power, to wealth and to reverence. He convinced people that his dream or irrationality was concrete reality and people started to believe it. Even today, thousands of individuals live on this same dupery.

Succession of failures

Scriptures like the Bible, with the plethora of praying and sacrificing, appear more like the story of a succession of failures to communicate. Failure of God to speak to Man clearly; failure of the Jews to recognize the Messiah; failure of Jesus to convince his fellow Jews (and the world at large) of his deity; failure of the Jews to communicate with God through prayer and sacrifice, especially at critical times such as the revelation of Jesus, and the Holocaust for example.

"But Nancy, what about the thousands of individuals who claim to have experienced miracles after prayer or sacrifice? Surely you can't just ignore them," says one of my guides. "I plan on returning to this well-known type of supernatural claim, but in due time. Allow me this indulgence, I reply."

"So then, what about considering God speaking to us", says one of my guides? "Maybe he does, or tries but, I have a hearing impediment, remember", I ask my religious guides? "Is there a way for Him to send us messages? Could it be that God would mysteriously consider these messages and in turn influence the course of human events or human individuals themselves? However small these direct influences, it would have to be by supernatural intervention. What type of supernatural influences (elements) could He then use?" "Let me explain it to you, but one question at a time", says my guide.

CHAPTER 4

CAN YOUR FRIEND SPEAK TO ME?

What have we learned?

We have learned that God, on the basis of His attributes, cannot possess certain attributes all at the same time because they are mutually exclusive. Despite the fact that He can potentially be omnipotent and omnibenevolent, He is either not simultaneously omniscient (doesn't know who suffers and prays) or He does not hear prayers at all. But then, if He does not hear prayers, He is not omnipotent. We are left with the feeling that prayer and ritual are not efficient means by which to communicate with this god. But there remains to see if God can speak to us somehow. Though we have just seen that there is no evidence that God hears and heeds our prayers, offerings and sacrifices, could he nevertheless intervene in our lives through mysterious spiritual elements? Is there a way for Him to speak to me? "So, you say that He can, then let's see", [speaking to my guide]. I may then heal from my hearing impairment.

Angels on high

In some religions, there exists certain 'messengers of god' commonly called Angels. The other names given to them are irrelevant here. These angels are at times considered as divine invisible spirits at others visible, materialized beings in the form most often of humans with wings. These mysterious messengers cannot be God himself for God is invisible. If we accept scriptures as evidence, God sent angels in ancient times as his representatives to appear to humans and to speak in his name [Psalm 103:20]. In accounts where it might seem that the Bible says that humans literally saw God, the context shows that God was represented by an angel or appeared by means of a vision. For example, God once spoke to Moses from a burning bush, and the Bible says that "Moses hid his face, because he was afraid to look at the true God." [Exodus 3:4, 6] Moses did not literally see God though, for the context shows that he actually saw "Jehovah's angel." [Exodus 3:2]. Similarly, when the Bible says that God "spoke to Moses face-to-face," it means that God conversed with Moses intimately, [Exodus 4:10, 11: 33:11]. Moses did not actually see God's face, for the information he received from God "was transmitted through angels" [Galatians 3:19; Acts 7:53]. Still, Moses' faith in God was so strong that the Bible described him as "seeing the One who is invisible" [Hebrews 11:27]. In the same way that he spoke to Moses, God is said to have communicated with Abraham through angels. Granted, a casual reading of the Bible might give the impression that Abraham literally saw God [Genesis 18:1, 33]. However, the context shows that the "three men" who came to Abraham were actually angels sent by God. Abraham recognized them as God's representatives and addressed them as if he were speaking directly to Jehovah [Genesis 18:2, 3, 22, 32; 19:1].

God has also appeared to humans through visions, or scenes presented to a person's mind. For instance, when the Bible says that Moses and other Israelites "saw the God of Israel," they really "saw a vision of the true God" [Exodus 24:9-11]. Likewise, the Bible sometimes says that prophets "saw Jehovah" [Isaiah 6:1; Daniel 7:9; Amos 9:1]. In each case, the context shows that they were given a vision of God rather than a direct view of him [Isaiah 1:1; Daniel 7:2; Amos 1:1] [7]

- No human has literally seen God; [Exodus 33:20; 1 John 4:12]
- "God is a Spirit," a form of life invisible to the human eye; [John 4:24; 1 Timothy 1:17]
- Angels, because they are spirit creatures, can communicate with God. [Mathew 18:10]
- Some humans who die will be able to see God; [Philippians 3:20, 21; 1John 3:21]

If they are spirits, invisible, immaterial 'beings', there is little one can do to try to find evidence of their existence. Science for sure has not invented the tools necessary to substantiate their existence. They remain in the realm of religious superstition until then. But, let us examine just a one among these chimeras for good measure.

Moroni, the angel

There are of course relatively well-known angel figures such as Moroni, who announces to a certain Joseph Smith in 1863, that some plates are hidden in a hill in New York State and that these plates relate the history of people who came to America as early as 300 to 400 A.D.

Now, Joseph Smith is a figure that really existed. He lived from 1805 to 1844 and is the founder of the original Mormon Religion; there are two churches now, at the last count. There is abundant, reliable information as to his tumultuous life and no historian would express a doubt as to his existence. It is not so much the figure that is to be considered here but the assertions of this founder. He is the only one to have seen this angel Moroni.

First, he announces that he has found gold and copper plates somewhere in New York state, that this angel told him where they were. Secondly, with the help of what he called "Urim and Thummim" (two stones set in a frame like a set of large spectacles), translates them from perhaps Greek, Aramaic, Reformed Egyptian hieroglyphs, into 268,163 English words. Yes, ladies and gentlemen, into English words, by a man, who had never studied any of the original languages attested to be engraved on the plates. Within a few months, behind a curtain, he dictates to a lonely secretary (at a time), 531 pages of stories from an original count of about 400 to 500 or fewer hieroglyphs; truly a miracle. That comes to about one full page of English text per hieroglyph; God truly works in mysterious ways. Surprisingly enough the 'translation' makes some sense even if too often it sounds very much like verses from the known Judeo-Christian scriptures. But a simple analysis of the story behind the moral and ethical verbiage does not stand a shadow of a chance of being historical truth and never will. There is to this date not the slightest historical evidence to the extravagant stories described in the Book of Mormon.

I have chosen this example because it brings us to the essential features of our quest for truth and evidence that we must use to analyze religion and its scriptures. To begin with, there are witnesses that have attested to the existence of the plates and sworn to the veracity of this miracle of translation by divine inspiration and a couple of stones. These witnesses are few and, one must add, not very reliable because too close to Smith himself and therefore of doubtful objectivity. They would never be admitted as accredited witnesses in any of today's modern courts. But despite this debate over the credibility and admissibility or not of such evidence in court, the contents of the translation (the Book of Mormon) destroy all authenticity of the plates whether or not the witnesses were honest as to their existence. By the way, they were perfectly incapable of reading the inscriptions and if they had seen plates, they could not attest to their inscribed content. This addition to the Old and New Testament is the translation of the plates that so conveniently were lost and have never been seen by anyone but the previously cited witnesses. It tells the story of people migrating from the Holy Land, across the Atlantic to the Americas, hundreds of years before Columbus and even hundreds of years before Christ. Too bad Columbus never heard about it. Should we re-write history and dethrone Columbus as discoverer of America based solely on these missing plates?

The Native Americans, according to this Book of Mormon, are nothing but the descendants of these Jewish people who colonized America before the beginning of the Christian era. Too bad today's Native Americans never knew this either and too bad they do not speak a word of Hebrew nor any remotely related language.

The book of Mormon basically says that the Native Americans that Columbus found were in fact the remnants of the original Jews that had abandoned God (Jesus, who appeared to them) and returned to evil ways and killed off all of the Good Jewish settlers. What is more, these people had built in North America, huge cities, used iron tools, metal coins, wheels and all that was known in Israel at the time, including animals (horses for ex.) that do not live in America until the arrival of Columbus. Not surprisingly, none of that civilization survived, not coins, not bones of domesticated middle-eastern animals, not even ruins. Though they are believers in the Bible as well, Mormons are technically speaking, heretics by virtue of the Orthodox Church if not the Catholic Church. The Book of Mormon is simply an offshoot of the Bible of very doubtful authenticity or validity to say the least. One must not accept anything at face value alone, especially invalidated testimony, as we shall see in a later chapter. Accepting Mormon Creed as it is written in the Book of Mormon is an incredible leap of faith indeed.

This brings us back to our angel or messenger of God. Why would a presumably intelligent angel, guard preciously the story of a whole culture of that importance for centuries, only to reveal the secret to an uneducated, clumsy fool, (he loses the plates), instead of revealing the plates to someone or some group with academic knowledge and education? In conclusion, this Moroni character is either a fool himself or simply a figment of Smith's imagination and a hoax. It is quite unconceivable that the Judeo-Christian-Islamic god would have sent such an incompetent angel and partaken in such a tall tale as this.

Either way, here again there is no tangible evidence of the existence of an angel.

Angels and dragons

If God meant for us to fly, he would have given us wings.
Unknown author

In a conventional image of a white-robed figure in human form with wings and a halo, some people picture a messenger of god. Native Americans for example would see messengers of god in the form of an eagle or other more rational and living being. However, some of these messengers can be of bad tidings as well, not to mention the so-called 'fallen angels', the most famous or infamous of which is of course Satan.

Flying men and women do not exist and have never existed without the help of a flying machine such as an airplane. A man with wings would be as helpless as one with elephant's ears, or elephants' feet. He could no more fly than a hippopotamus can climb trees. A flying man would be as impossible and ridiculous as a flying cow. Why do boats have a keel? Why don't we simply build floating houses or floating skyscrapers? Why don't airplanes look like flying houses? Because of something called aerodynamics and hydrodynamics. Imagine taking the wings off a Boeing 707 and replacing them with two wooden framed paper kites. Then imagine trying to make it fly. That is roughly as close to the image of a Dragon you would get as they are pictured in medieval representations; huge beasts with dinky wings. Angels are pictured with bigger wings and feathers than a bird but they have no more flight muscles and proper articulations than a kite-winged Boeing 707, nor the strength to take off and maintain flight.

So where do these images of a supernatural human being, either good or bad, with a white robe, with wings and a halo come from? And what credit can we give to these depictions? First of all the biological and physiological considerations of such a creature easily show the obsolete and dysfunctional nature of such wings. They can only be myths or legends, chimeras, fabulous, impossible creatures of someone's imagination and irrationality. The only back-boned animals that have wings are birds and bats and some rare squirrels. In geologic times Pterodactyls had wings and yet they are not considered having been angels simply because they seem hideous to us and have no human form. There is no skeleton in any tomb or in the fossil record that shows and proves that an angel, a human with wings, has ever existed.

If an angel is supposed to be a supernatural being, it doesn't need wings to fly. If it has magical, divine, supernatural powers it should most cleverly fly without wings. If it is a spirit of some sort, capable of taking on human form, like a ghost of sorts, it needs not any wings. It is probably 'Ethereal' in nature, bodiless, immaterial and thus one would genuinely infer, lighter than air; once again, no need for wings.

Does all this mean that angels, as messengers of god, do not exist? No, but if they do, it is certainly not in the form of winged human figures. They would be the perfect two-way accessibility to God. Like your invisible friend they have attributes, listed in all scriptures, some of which are; they have spirit bodies (Revelation 4:8), they are immortal (2 Thessalonians 1:7-10) and yet they eat food (Numbers 22:35), they can be visible or invisible (Revelation 8:13 & John 20:12), they can travel at incredible speed (Matthew 18:10). Just like with your invisible friend, some of these attributes are incompatible or at least contradictory: Why for example would an immortal being need to eat or drink.

Unfortunately, just like the other modes of intervention, there is to this day no substantiated, relevant, objective evidence for such spirits; nothing acceptable as evidence in a courtroom or as scientific evidence either. Remember, I am keeping the intervention by miracles for a little later.

By now my guides are burning to shout out, "I have a book sent to us by my invisible friend himself that says who He is and what he wants!" All institutionalized religions claim to know what (or who) is out there. Each religion claims that it has "absolute" truth about some god it knows. By the way, there is no such thing as an absolute truth. Something is either true, or it is false. Adding the superlative "absolute", does not change anything to its state. There is no such thing as a half-truth or a half-false statement.

"So, all right, let's have a look at your invisible friend's messages."

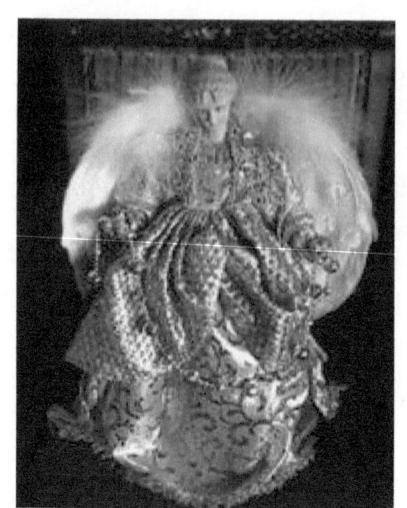

CHAPTER 5

YOUR FRIEND'S GREATEST MESSAGE

Messages called scriptures

Whether or not such things as Angels exist or not, the fact is that those who see and hear their friend say that He offers writings known as scriptures, or sacred writings that attest to his miracles and his intentions. These people refer to these scriptures as the foundations for their religion. They say that they are the very "Word of God". As a non-believer, I can say that it appears obvious that they were not written by this invisible friend with plume in hand since He has no hands; He's immaterial. However, He is supernatural and eventually omnipotent, if this is not incompatible with another attribute, in which case He could whisper the text to a person who would then write it down. Therefore, we can only focus on the result of this trick, in other words the texts themselves. But before we look at them per se, we can honestly ask what type of texts could we expect to see emanating from this supernatural friend? Remember that hearing voices is not normal or natural and cannot be accepted as evidence in a court of law (thank goodness).

Here is the core of the subject. If what religion claims to know about God is contained in its scriptures, then we must focus on their contents. However, I have no intention in indulging in the study of these writings any more than is necessary for punctual references and essential issues; no intention of interpreting them. As far as I am concerned, they have no intrinsic value until they can be corroborated. Besides, all three institutionalized Judeo-Christian-Islamic religions have their own set of scriptures. We must analyze them from the outside looking in (not from an apologetic view) to determine if they are valid and authentic in other words logical, rational and I would even add, useful not to mention intelligent and worthy of the greatest mind there is.

Godly simplifications

Let us start for example with two simplified hypothetical scenarios that follow the essential message of Christianity (monotheistic hypothesis) as it has been exposed over the last 2000 years, at least, to see if it is worthy of the most intelligent mind in the universe; this is a first scenario in a short series.

Summarily:
- First phase; God (the Christian one) creates the Universe, the Earth, animals, plants and Man who is an imperfect being (we will return to this attribute later so keep this in mind).
- Second phase; God decrees divine laws, rules and commandments (heretofore called laws for short) to help Man live a moral and happy life.
- Third phase; the very first man, Adam (in the literal sense), and very first woman, Eve (also in the literal sense), break the very first law.
- Fourth phase; God says to Man and Woman, "you did not obey my command therefore I must punish you both" (for the honor and the principle, we presume). "From this day on a breach of my laws will be called a Sin" (God invents the sin).
- Fifth phase; God says that he gave Man a choice (a vague and disingenuous form of Free Will) but he did not heed; being given the choice to walk 10 miles home or take a shortcut of 5 miles by jumping off a 200-foot cliff is not a very honest or genuine choice.
- Sixth phase; now humans must pay a penalty of infinite consequences; first, man will die instead of being immortal (Genesis), he and his mate will suffer and toil for the rest of their lives and his children and all of mankind will suffer for eternity. But, good news, He has a plan for each human.
- Seventh phase; God informs Man that there are many other laws he must now abide by and that some of them are not only under penalty of death but also under penalty of eternal damnation of the soul (mortal sins of the soul).
- Eighth phase; God creates a Guilt-forever-syndrome in which each human must toil to stay within the limits of good and evil (subjective concept with blurred boundaries), wondering if they are

doing the right thing or not, incessantly, and living in the obsession of perpetual repentance (prayers, sacrifices, rituals…).
- Ninth phase; after thousands of years, this god decides that he has been a little rough, so he decides to show humans how things should be done (or should have been done). He sends himself in the form of his one and only son (incarnation) to a sacrifice; not to a beheading (quick and humane death) or a poisoning (quick and humane death) or a push off a 200-foot cliff (quick and humane death), but the most barbaric, brutal, inhumane death that Man has ever invented (Crucifixion). Does this remind you of anyone (Machiavel, Sade, Dracula…)?
- Tenth phase; God proposes that anyone who would condone the murder of his son (aka himself) would be pardoned of all sin and possibly admitted into heaven (a place where one relives a second time but happily) if they acknowledge Christ as their savior (Salvation); what a marvelous and ingenious gift to mankind (satire).
- Eleventh phase; God has already prepared two superb resorts for the others who choose (Free Will) not to accept this massacre as a form of Redemption; one is purgatory, the other is Hell where souls are roasted forever with refinement and attention by his henchman, Satan, who takes great pride and pleasure in satisfying his master.
- Twelfth phase; If you make the "choice" of phase 10, you get to go back to phase 8 for the remainder of your earthly life.

Conclusions: What a loving and merciful deity; the intricate superfluities only add to his glory (satire). My religious guides continue to remind me that His love and mercy are unconditional despite evidence to the contrary. Religion states that this is why we need this god in order for redemption, and for salvation from something this god invented; sin, a sort of metaphysical leash.

Now let us try in the same way a second simplified hypothetical scenario that still follows the essential message of Christianity; merciful, creative, all-powerful and all-intelligent god, etc.

- First phase; God (the Christian one) creates the Universe, the Earth, animals, plants and Man… (Remember he is imperfect).

- Second phase; God creates guidelines to help Man live a moral and happy life and reveals these guidelines through divine inspiration (whatever that is).
- Third phase; God gives Man Free Will, in other words the choice between following his guide-lines or not following them, with a simple warning that Man may become very miserable if he does not.
- Fourth phase; some humans choose to follow God's advice and they are for the most part happy and moral.
- Fifth phase; some humans choose not to follow God's guidelines; as a result, many of them are miserable and immoral: They reap what they sow.
- Sixth phase; God intervenes to reward those who followed his guidelines through gifts, blessings, praise and possibly an eternal life of the soul somewhere (concept of heaven).
- Seventh phase; many more humans choose to follow the guidelines in order to obtain the same type of rewards.

Conclusions: In this scenario, God does not punish anyone. He appears as a good and loving god who allows free will and does not threaten anyone. He offers rewards instead of punishments in order to help Man become more reasonable, moral and happy. Which of the two scenarios would you have chosen if you were this all-intelligent deity?

But, my guides remind me that Christianity affirms that 'complexities are necessary to authenticate the interventions and intentions of our God'.

Omniscience and communication

Omniscience is the state of knowing everything that there is to know. This can only mean that God would be capable of perfect rationality, perfect logic and perfect intelligence. This means that He is in essence capable of clarity, coherence, purpose and technical prowess. His actions and messages should be the epitome of style, clarity, usefulness and devoid of ambiguity, bias, equivocalness and mundane pettiness. In that respect, we can compare God with an alien of a highly advanced civilization. "Now, just a moment!" says my guide. "God is smarter than the smartest alien ever"; and I would do not defer. "Let us just for the sake of the discussion, and our query, focus for a moment on what might happen if such an alien came into contact with us here on Earth" I retort.

So, here is a short series of food-for-thought scenarios on this topic:

Imagine, in a first scenario, that we have been contacted by a highly advanced alien civilization on a distant planet whose sun will explode within a few weeks. They want to share their accumulated knowledge with us before their planet is destroyed. Imagine also that you are their head scientist. You have been given the responsibility for choosing the nature of the information that will be shared.

You only have about a week to transmit the information but the planet could explode sooner than expected. What information will you send and in what order of priority will you send it? Choose only about 10 proprietary subjects.

Take a few moments to think it over and perhaps make a list.

A Second scenario: Imagine this time, that you are the head of the Science committee in charge of sending our accumulated knowledge to a distant alien intelligence we have contacted and that it is our planet Earth which is dying. You have a week to send as much data as possible knowing that the planet could explode sooner than expected.

A measure of our intelligence as a species might be calibrated on the quality and the amount of information we could be able or willing to share with an advanced alien civilization capable of visiting us physically or capable through telecommunications of contacting us. Their capability of contacting us or visiting our planet would be an indication of advanced technology. Our messages and knowledge would perhaps place us in the dark-ages of science from their point of view, so do your best.

Among the subjects listed below, which ones would you send in order of priority, if you could only choose from this list?
- The Encyclopedia Britannica.
- The winners of the Golden Globe Awards of the past 10 years.
- A complete set of nursery rhymes and fairy tales.
- The past 50 years of discoveries in Physics and Astrophysics.
- The list of Nobel Prize winners of the last 60 years.
- The past 50 years of research in Biology and Genetics.

- The complete King James version of the Bible, the complete Quran, and the complete Book of Mormon.
- A multi-volume compendium of the history of a specific country of your choice.
- The expounded Theory of Evolution both historical (Darwinian) and Modern.
- A description of the Vatican and other holy sites on our planet.

You can see that this exercise helps to give us a more humble and objective outlook on our priorities on Earth.

Here is a third scenario in which you are god (take your pick).

You have just created a planet (Earth) among billions of others. You are almighty, but fathoms out beyond the frontiers of this universe. You have populated the Earth with at least one intelligent species. The individuals of this species have life spans of a split second in comparison to your scale of time. You are extremely busy, but you wish to see them thrive and live intelligently, in peace, and happiness and be the healthiest they can. You have decided to create optimal conditions for their welfare and survival. What conditions will you create for them and in what order of priority? Take a break and think it over and perhaps make a list.

Now what do you think of the following list?
- A titanium plated skeleton to help them from breaking their bones.
- Give claws and fur to help them defend themselves and survive the cold.
- Temperatures varying from -15 degrees F to + 110 degrees F in as many regions as possible with seasonal variations.
- Predators to eat them and weed out the old and less fit.
- An atmosphere containing oxygen in quantities compatible with life.
- A mechanical heart to allow them to live long prosperous lives.
- Enough easy to capture animals to sustain them.
- Trees and wood for fire and making shelters.
- Stones for building shelters and making tools.
- Germs and diseases to weed out the less fit.

Now consider this fourth and last scenario where you are god (take your pick). You have just created a planet (Earth) among billions of others with intelligent beings. You have decided to send them a message (or even a series of messages) to help them survive and organize their societies. What messages will you send them and in what order of priority? Take a break and think it over.

Now what do you think of the following list?
- A manual on how to make tools, starting with stone ones.
- A manual on how a man can live in a whale.
- A manual on human rights.
- A manual on why women should not be allowed as priests or equals to men.
- A manual on how to build an Ark.
- A manual on how to recognize forbidden fruits.
- A manual on how to make fire.
- A manual on how to name animals.
- A manual of 10 rules to follow for societal living, some of which repeat themselves.
- A manual on how to make a wheel and use it.
- A manual on how to destroy your enemies; burning, stoning, drowning, blowing horns to demolish walls, etc.

A litmus test

These four scenarios are a reflection upon the extent to which intelligence is present in the universe in the form of alien civilizations or even in the form of a god or gods. If aliens could send us scientific, let alone intelligent, rational, logical, useful, constructive, concise information, just as we would attempt to do for our honor, think of what an omniscient God should be able to do by analogy.

"There are important messages for us in the scriptures", say my guides. "Here is a passage in Corinthians for example, read it and you will see". So I comply and come back to say, "Can I be honest with you"? I ask. "Yes of course", is their answer.

"Well, amid sordid, complex, fait-diver imbroglios and a petty mundane gossip file, I finally stumbled across what a particular scholar or priest might find essential; it reads like this, "If you hang out with bad guys, you will become a bad guy". Now in today's world something as common sense as this would seem an insult to any person of normal intelligence; this is why I won't even give the coordinates of the passage. If you want to read it, see for yourself how much fun it is trying to find it. It appears that the essentials are strewn and buried among an entanglement, a web of incredibly mundane, petty, boring and almost insane stories and tons of he-said, she-said local trivia involving unknown people with tortured minds. In any other circumstances, such a collection of hog-wash would be considered the work of at least one gossip queen or even one village idiot."

Already, it does not speak well for the clarity of mind of this universal brain. For example, it would help if there was a logical progression of events, lessons, examples… that one could easily understand and follow… but, there is none. What use is a book of this presumed importance, without an Index, a Bibliography, something to help the reader through? There is not one mathematical, prepositional, practical, lexical, numerical, alphabetical… index anywhere. Apparently, the information is so important that it is almost impossible to find without a doctorate in so-called theology, and without theologians, thus giving some legitimacy to the necessity of these humbugs.

"Now Nancy, you are being injurious here", say my guides. "You will understand why I say this in a later chapter, so allow me this extreme for once", I Answer.

So then, just how sound is the message from your invisible friend? As illustrated in the last two previous scenarios, a measure, a litmus test of the intelligence and the omniscience of a hypothetical universal god could be the nature of messages sent to us by this deity or the nature of His creation. But, we can already clearly see that what these scriptures tell us of God is contradictory, confusing, belittling, and far from the depictions that churches wantonly diffuse of a sort of super-god, an almighty deity capable of anything and everything especially of clarity and leadership. They are not useful for agriculture or for construction of homes, cities or governments, even less for mathematics, physics, chemistry, astronomy, etc.

In the next few chapters we are going to analyze the claims put forth by religions as to the origin of their knowledge of a universal deity and the authenticity of the evidence they pretend to have through these messages (Scriptures) from God. The most important question being, "how reliable are these scriptures"? After all, as we shall see later, they had to be copied and this is where trouble starts because to make copies, someone must copy by hand and know the language of the original especially if a translation is necessary.

The authentication of religion is linked to the reliability of its books. This leads us to a more focused analysis of these divinely inspired writings or scriptures. Here are some of the questions we will add to those already asked:

- Should we take scriptures literally?
- Do scriptures contain myth and legend?
- Do scriptures contain errors of transcription (copy)?
- Are scriptures viable historical records?
- Are scriptures viable scientific references (formation of the Earth, the stars, the cosmos)?
- Are scriptures metaphorical and mystic interpretations of the world?

"My first impression is that translating scriptures into your spoken language, whichever it is, doesn't visibly (no pun intended) help much since you still have to go to church regularly to have someone read it and interpret it for you and tell you what it is really intended to say; decidedly this god is not the literary genius he is made out to be and certainly not the greatest mind of the universe," I say to my guides.

"Well Nancy, we are here to help you see straight in all of this, just be patient and not so systematically critical," says one of my guides.

"OK," I reply, "let's do it".

CHAPTER 6

SO YOUR FRIEND HAS A BOOK?

How reliable is your friend's book?

"That which can be asserted without evidence can also be dismissed without evidence."
Christopher Hitchens in *God is not great*

As we all know, all of the Judeo-Christian-Islamic religions call what is basically the same god by different names, aliases or nicknames. This is something that should trouble any and all believers. Each will tell you they know this god better than all the others because they have his words in a book, their book. This is where Science with critical thinking and rational analysis, comes in to help set things straight. Science can focus on essentially three criteria; authenticity, validity, and authority of scriptures.

- Authenticity is linked to historicity
- Validity is linked to the amount of veracity and depends on the evidence, credentials, facts, data, and records related to their book.
- Authority is linked to the amount of justification and corroboration of the two previous criteria.

Just how much of scripture is true and inerrant? If the answer is "all of it, *in extensor*", then we are faced with a simple experiment. This experiment consists of analyzing the Bible or any other scriptures and researching the presence of but one element that cannot be true in the sense of not being admissible in a court of law or even contrary to scientific probability. If this element or event casts but a shadow of doubt on the scripture's veracity then the entire work becomes doubtful. This is one of those keystones that when pulled from the forbidden wall of religion causes all above it to crash. The premise here is that if 99.9% of the Bible or any other scripture is true, it's not enough to eliminate the doubt cast by the 0.1% false or doubtful element. The Torah and the Qur'an are not immune to this form of examination and contain their own dose of myth and legend. "But," says my guide, "this is a standard of measurement far too extreme, don't you think?" "Let's not forget that it is you and your religion which claim that you know God and that the Scriptures are His Word, the word of an all-intelligent God", I reply. "Christopher Hitchens has written, eloquently, that extraordinary claims, demand extraordinary evidence, and I would add extraordinary standards of measure. Does this appear fair enough to you?" I ask.

They all consent to this argument.

Who believes in Noah's ark?

The Protestants believe that Noah, forewarned by god, built a boat into which he had taken seven other persons and either twos or sevens of every animal in the world and fed them for sixty-one days or three hundred and sixty-five days (depending on the chapter), all other creatures on earth being destroyed. This story was accepted as a myth by the scientific community as early as the 19th century for several reasons, one of which we will consider.

Churches such as the Protestant ones are sometimes willing to admit to some misinterpretations due to the imperfections of the men who translated and transcribed the scriptures. But when they admit the presence of legends and myths, it puts once again the whole edifice to doubt. Where does one draw the line? Where then does truth in the texts begin, and legend or myth end? Besides, theoretically, the Roman Catholic Church (or by primacy, the Eastern Orthodox Church) is the only authority on the Bible, period; all the rest is heresy.

Build a new ark

An interesting experiment would be to build a new ark and in Kentucky [8] one man has built one. With the help of philanthropists the construction, with modern technology, of a new ark to the specifications of the Bible has been accomplished. It could be manned by four men and four women and loaded with as many animal couples as possible and food. Modern shipyards can handle such a vessel and it could be brought out into the Atlantic or Pacific oceans for a test run. No one would object to equipping it with a GPS, two-way radios, life jackets and lifeboats for safety. This would nail the case. Unfortunately it sits on dry land. What is worse is that it is electrified (modern technology), something that was not available to Noah. It would be literally impossible for 8 people to feed animals, and circulate in this dark cave of a ship (no windows) with an oil lamp in one hand and a bale of hay in the other. Not to mention that the risk of setting the ship on fire would have been too great.

It would have been interesting to see everyone's reaction if Bill Nye the Science Guy [9] who had visited it had asked his host to turn off all of the electric lights once they were in the belly of the ship; that would have been a clincher.

The Noachian Paradox

Let me go straight to the point. Let's admit for the sake of the discussion that such an event really occurred. Imagine for a moment that you free all of these animals after the flood, it is impossible that they would all find their way, across oceans, continents, mountains, rivers and thousands of miles to the lands where they are known today (except for birds perhaps). As early as 1753, everyone understood, and even the Pope, that most animal species, if not all, had not migrated from the Bible-lands, a common source in Armenia, but had originated in situ, in other words in the regions where they are still known today for the most part. The essential element of the Noachian flood story arises after the flood when it reaches land; here is why it never happened.

Now when everything had dried up, some long time later (370 to 400 days) [Genesis chap. 8:13&14, not to mention Genesis chap. 8: 5, 6, 7, 10, 12], Noah's menagerie finally came to town, or rather to land. He finally let everything loose. Can you imagine how hungry these things were, especially the Giants, Cyclops and the Dinosaurs, the Mammoths, the Mastodons, the Glyptodonts, and the lions...? They were famished.

In 1777, Eberhardt Zimmermann [10], an early zoologist, published an interesting and little-known tract, *Specimen Zoologiae Geographicae Quadrupedum*, in which he ridiculed the idea that only one pair of each kind of animal, was in the Ark [11](see also; *The Secular Ark* by Janet Browne, 1983). After such a prolonged sojourn in the ship, upon their release, the last pair of lions would eat the last pair of sheep, soon followed by the last pair of goats, and other herbivores in one quick succession. Finally, even the lions would die of starvation after having eaten everything in sight. Even if some got away there would be no predators like lions left for us to see today. Even then, it remained to explain how these few survivors would have gotten to where they now live by crossing continents, rivers and even oceans. This same analysis is true with seven of each kind. In finale, Noah tries to save the animals of Earth only to lead them to a certain death by starvation and extinction; this is the Noachian Paradox.

A layer of humans in the mud

If a universal flood did wipe out millions of animals and thousands of humans, where then is the layer of hardened mud that should contain the bones of these humans and of these Dinosaurs, Mammoths, giants, and various other now extinct animals that the flood killed in one swift swoop? I don't mean that they should be lying side by side within 10, 100 feet or even 100 miles of one another, but in the same geological strata, dating from the same period of time. There is none. Why? Because the last dinosaurs for example died out some 64 million years before the first human skeleton appeared in the fossil record. This is another reason why Noah's flood never happened.

There is scientific evidence all over the world of various floods. These floods took place in different parts of the world, at very different periods of time. But there is no geological evidence what so ever for a universal flood, having affected the whole world within a time frame of one year (or even more) and especially at the hypothesized time period suggested by most proponents of such an event.

Some recent finds suggest that there may have been a devastating flood in the Balkans in and around the biblical time mentioned for Noah's flood. If this is true and geologically established one day, this will only go to prove that Noah's flood would have been a geographically localized event with few animals and, once again, not universal.

Consequence for Jesus

Religion tells us that Jesus Christ was an eyewitness to the Flood. He had a pre-human existence (Proverbs 8:30, 31). He was a spirit creature in heaven during the Flood. In the Bible Jesus is quoted as saying that "just as the days of Noah were, so the presence of the Son of Man will be. For as they were in those days before the flood, ... until the day that Noah entered into the ark; and they took no note until the flood came and swept them all away, so the presence of the Son of Man will be". (Matthew 24:37-39)

The frightening thing here is that if these people apply this logic to its end, then they have just proven that Jesus was not really the Son of God they believe he is. If the Flood, as it appears to Catholic religion and most true scientists, never existed, then Jesus could never have witnessed it in his pre-human state. The fact that he speaks of it is only because he read about it himself in Genesis which we presume he had studied. Jesus then is but a man, not a god. The corollary of this fact is that Jesus is not the Messiah and the authenticity and authority of the Christian Religion is obliterated. It contains its own destructive elements. But, what if the ark is but a metaphor, a myth after all? Jesus (of the scriptures) speaks of it as a reality.

What have we learned?

One important conclusion can be made from this analysis: Not only do the scriptures contain at least 0.1% of myth and legend, in reality they contain much more such as Jonas and the fish (or whale), the legendary Moses, the adulteress woman and Jesus, Joshua stopping the Sun, etc.; more than we have time for in this book. Even at this point we can already clearly say that the Bible cannot be considered in its entirety as a reliable, literal and accurate source of truth on past events, at least not to 100%.

In his *Deceptions and Myths of the Bible*, Lloyd Graham, whoever he may be in real life, demonstrates that he has a more than average knowledge of the Biblical Scriptures. He is demonstrably a scholar in his own right though some argue that he is not a scholar for lack of an official, accredited title or diploma as if one cannot do a scholarly analysis without one. Though he hides behind his pen name and his anonymity, he has seen and proven beyond a doubt that the Bible is an accumulation of myths and legends which he highlights judiciously, one by one, in his voluminous publication. However, he stops short for some unknown reason, of taking the next inevitable step of declaring it a work without worth in matters of the knowledge of a god. Instead, he gets caught up, like most scholars before him, in the maze of entrapments and corridors that lead him in circles to interpretations of yet other interpretations; his essential conclusion (Chapter 25, page422)is that the Bible's texts are the results of a deliberate misinterpretation of Pagan myths and legends, so he indulges in yet his own interpretations, just to add and aggravate the abundance of such useless endeavors... since the bottom line is that they have therefore (whatever their meaning) no value, no authority, and no authenticity in matters of the god whose 'word' they are supposed to be. So, he leaves us hanging on the edge of a cliff with the question, "Is there anything left of the Bible that is not doubtful"? In other words, just what is the remaining value of the so-called testimony in scriptures? Is there any truth in scriptures at all? Is communicating with god a hoax?

In retrospect, for those who know them, scriptures appear to be poor examples of rationality, logic and usefulness. There is an obvious disconnect between the contents of these books and the omniscience of a divine universal God. These scriptures are tortuous stories that are demonstrably in constant need of reinterpretations which religion has been contending with for centuries and which continue to divide churches and denominations. Why would an all-intelligent deity send us useless myths and legends even if they contain some moral teachings and not useful information for our survival as a species?

At this point I want to highlight an essential element of religion. If we have learned anything it's that scriptural religion can only rely on its scriptures for truth; the scriptures are the basic principles, the foundations. This means that a religion can only be fundamentalist (etymologically) in other words strictly based on its sacred writings. These writings can only be true or false, there cannot be any other position or they lose their value. But, over the last 2000 years they have been interpreted over and over again and mostly cherry-picked to the point of no longer having any authenticity or intrinsic value evidenced in the plethora of new churches and denominations that have reduced the scriptures to a handful of selected principles, quotes, and pages.

According to the two-volume *World Christian Encyclopedia* (Barrett, Kurian, and Johnson; Oxford University Press: February 2016), World Christianity consists of 6 major ecclesiastic-cultural blocs, divided into 300 major ecclesiastical traditions, composed [*sic*] of over 33,000 distinct denominations in 238 countries (Vol. I, p. 16). The WCE then goes on to break down "world Christianity" into the following broad categories:
- Independents: 22,000 denominations
- Protestants: 9000 denominations
- Marginal: 1600 denominations

- Orthodox: 781 denominations
- Catholics: 242 denominations
- Anglicans: 168 denominations

There are many other sources of contended numbers, but this in itself is a blatant admission that these writings have no intrinsic divine value. There should be only one church, one denomination if such writings were indisputably true.

But, in all honesty, religions and my religious guides tell me that there is more to the message (scriptures) and there are numerous witnesses that attest to the stories that they contain. We must then, in all objectivity, analyze the historicity, the validity and the authenticity of the rest of this message(s) from the greatest mind there is.

CHAPTER 7

THE VALUE OF WRITTEN DOCUMENTS

If it's written, it's true

If religion had remained purely orally transmitted, two consequences would have ensued. If all those who had the oral knowledge were to succumb, the religion would be lost. If the holders of knowledge were to be suspected of falsifying their knowledge of god(s), if their powers were to be questioned, the validity of the religion would collapse and people would go in search of a better one. This latter consequence has most probably been the case of countless primitive religions, replaced over and over again by more powerful ones, by choice or by conquest. Early institutionalized monotheistic religions in particular, soon understood these risks and with the advent of writing, they soon wrote what was then easily presentable (to those who didn't write or read), as being dictated by a god himself. If god dictated it, it is true in many believers' minds.

How much credence can we give a written story, especially one as old as the scriptures? We have just seen that several stories (Noah, Jonas, Moses and more) are more than doubtful and can only be myths or legends even with a small nucleus of truth. It appears already that the scriptures contain many texts that can only have been included by literate humans and not a god because He would have known better. The scriptures cannot have been dictated entirely by an omniscient (and/or omnipotent) god. This is perhaps one of the most difficult realities religious people must face. Therefore, it is only legitimate that we analyze the validity and value of these texts many of which are allegedly from witnesses to events.

I believe in Nemo and Oz

Most people in America and the western world have seen the movie version of the book "the Wizard of OZ" by Lyman Frank Baum, read it or heard of it. The same is true of Jules Verne's "20,000 leagues under the Sea". Let's make just a simple analysis of these two big classics. Both make mention of places that really exist or have existed: Kansas, Paris, London and many more. Does this make them geography or history reference books? No of course not. Both describe natural phenomena such as tornadoes, ocean creatures, volcanic eruptions and the like. Does this make them reference books for Meteorology, Geology, or Oceanography? No of course not. Both make reference to people with simple common names such as Dorothy, Emma, Nemo, and so on. Does this make these people real? No of course not.

Quite obviously, if someone were to discover a birth certificate of a Dorothy-of-Oz or a Dorothy-of-Kansas or of a Captain Nemo-of-the-Nautilus, then we would have some serious reconsideration to make as to the authenticity of such stories. Nevertheless, on another register, the authors of these books were real people; we have records of their birth dates, parents, school diplomas and many other documents that attest to their reality. Not only were they well educated, and well versed in their mother tongues but they had credentials as writers and scholars; there is no doubt as to their sincerity or honorableness even if their books are works of fiction.

An individual taking these works of fiction on faith alone could voluntarily believe they are true even in the face of all of the documents attesting to their fantasy. Could you imagine meeting someone who would proclaim that there is a Witch-of-the-West, one of the east and so on, based solely on the Wizard of Oz? Imagine this person claiming, "Dorothy said... I believe it". "If you sincerely believe, you too can be transported to Kansas by knocking your heels together." The same can be done with "20,000 leagues under the sea"; "Nemo said... I believe it." This is no different from the apparent dysfunctional behavior of people who quote scripture without *a priori* establishing its veracity.

Elusive accuracy

Before Man invented the writing of historical events, they were transmitted orally from one generation to the other. What precedes history is of course what archaeologists call Prehistory because there is no written record for any events. When Man invented writing and had a support for it that could last, such as stones, clay tablets and papyrus, it became possible to keep an ongoing record of events. We teach our children historical events because they link us to our past, our ancestors. History of a family is important to give children a sense of belonging to a group of people who are related. History of the world ties us into the bonds that unite people of a same country and consequently of course to all of humanity. But how do historians determine the truth from the legend and the myth? Just how can we know what is correct in ancient writings?

Recording events is not enough. These recordings must be corroborated. If someone writes about himself using flattery and exaggeration, we may get the wrong impression about their role in society and their influence in all sorts of political and social affairs. If the record has been written by several independent chroniclers of preferably different opinions and viewpoints, then it is easier to determine just how much the record is accurate and objective. History is a matter of accuracy and veracity.

There are numerous texts that have survived centuries and have given modern historians ample access to ancient events and figures of human history. The list of these chroniclers and also of the anonymous writings that create a spectrum of documents going as far back as prehistory is too long to detail here of course. Just how precise and credible are these texts? How can we know what is true and what is fiction? One of the first great medieval explorers of History focused on accuracy was Francesco Petrarch (1304 -1374 A.D.) [12].

The pioneer of modern historical criticism was Lorenzo Valla (1407 – 1457) [13]. His writings called *Annotations on the New Testament* among others were printed in 1505 and fueled the fire lit at the Reformation (Luther 1517). Lorenzo Valla was convicted of heresy, on eight counts, by the Inquisition and condemned to burn at the stake, after demonstrating that the *Apostle's Creed* could not have been composed by the twelve Apostles; [see, *The Discoverers*, by Daniel J. Boortin, 1983].[14]

The value of historical texts

The Greek epic poet Homer who lived in the 9th century B.C. is reputed the author (according to legend) of the Iliad and the Odyssey which we all have heard of if not read in school. The story that he tells of the Trojan wars is truly an epic. The existence of a city that may have been Troy was discovered by archaeologists and what is more was with the help of descriptions and clues in the writings themselves. Archaeologists have found evidence that this presumed Troy was the victim of wars and possibly a siege at one time but, the evidence found may only be circumstantial as yet. Even so, this does not mean that everything that Homer (or another author) wrote is the truth and nothing but the truth. It certainly doesn't mean that all of the characters and supernatural beings (Cyclops, mermaids, etc.) truly existed. It does not mean that Poseidon and the palette of other gods described in the book are real. Even if other stories have been found that mention such similar characters and supernatural beings, no acceptable evidence of the existence of such beings has ever been found. Now of course if one day, archaeologists uncovered the remains of a cyclops or a mermaid, then perhaps would we have to seriously review these writings? Moreover, perhaps we would have to consider taking up the worship of Greek gods?

Therefore, however old a written text may be, it is not because it is written that it is necessarily the truth or all of the truth. Historians, scientists, judges, juries all need acceptable, corroborated, unequivocal, and substantiated evidence to determine the truth in any circumstance, in any event whether historical or contemporary. For example, there is no doubt in the mind of any self-respecting historian that Moses is a legendary figure though the Old Testament speaks of him as a real person.

Establishing authentication

When Caesar writes about Caesar how much of what he says of himself is true, especially when he is trying to gain prestige during his own lifetime? Fortunately, other people have chronicled the events and the people he wrote about. These other chroniclers are not as biased as he is and this gives us a better view of the true situations and events. When someone writes about himself or someone else, however close, without anyone else to chronicle what they say about him or her, we can legitimately doubt the veracity of the text. What is particularly difficult to authenticate is what someone may have said orally to someone else. If only one of these interlocutors keeps a diary or soon after the discussion reports the words exchanged in written form by letter, there is then an authentication possible. If known and objective chroniclers of biblical times were to have written texts telling a similar or identical story to that which is found in our earliest biblical manuscripts, there would be corroboration, but there is none.

For example, can the Bible be considered a Science reference? There is little or no scientific information (worth mentioning) in the Bible that can be of any use to modern Science. It therefore is certainly not a

Science book. Besides it is replete with supernatural events and Science deals with natural events. What then of History? The Egyptians, Maya, Inca, Aztecs, and many other cultures made numerous mentions of exact calendar dates often based on elaborate astronomical observations and literally carved in stone. But, there is nowhere to be found, in the entire Bible the slightest corroborated calendar date, whatever the calendar standard. This is rather detrimental to authenticity, obviously. This is one of the primary reasons why the Bible can't be considered a History book. The Bible reads like a novel and not like a documentary of any precision no matter how much hermeneutic is applied to it. It is a hodgepodge of myths, legends and mundane, petty gossip.

One important conclusion comes from our analysis: In order to establish the truth about an event, historians need documents from at least one objective source that gives accurate and verifiable geographical, chronological and historical references; the more reliable the author and the more sources of objective corroborating documents the better. So far in our quest we have not encountered any. We must pursue our investigation.

What do we have left, Philosophy, Metaphysics and the like? Here at least we can agree that it fits in these categories. In consequence, it can only be taken on faith for it has no valid facts. There is little that can be usefully authenticated in the Bible other than place names, some fleeting events and cultural traits. Whether or not a man called Jesus, the Christ really existed or not is actually a completely different issue.

Millions and Billions

What then is the value of a witness, or even millions of witnesses if there is no objective evidence? The number of Christians, who have believed in Jesus and the Bible as an inerrant collection of testimonies over the past 2000 year is irrelevant. Dozens of so-called witnesses, even hundreds or thousands, without objective corroborating evidence or objective corroborating witnesses (unbiased) is not viable, acceptable testimony, at least not in a court of law. It is not because millions upon millions or even billions of people have for 2000 years thought or believed that Jesus was real, that he was. It is not because millions upon millions of people, including myself, have thought and believed that Santa Claus was real, that he is.

The existence of a group of texts, that we now call the New Testament, some of which were refuted by the early Church itself (Apocrypha) because not in line with the agenda of the Church or just plain contradictory, makes of these scriptures a hodge-podge of various texts chosen by the Church of the 4th century AD with no particular and admissible validity. Even if they are representative of the original whole, the question of their accuracy and authenticity remains.

Quoting erroneous texts

This brings us to the question of the origins of the scriptures that remain today in most institutionalized religions. In his groundbreaking, book Misquoting Jesus (2005), Bart D. Ehrman [15] brings scholarly proof that the texts so dear to Christians for example derive from originals that have not been found and that may never be found. What is more, the New Testament (NT) translations of various authors have flaws beyond belief (no pun intended) because they are based on wrong texts.

Bart D. Ehrman chairs the Department of Religious Studies at the University of North Carolina at Chapel Hill. He is an authority on the history of the New Testament, the early church and the life of Jesus. He states, (not verbatim), "... the translations of the NT, available to most English readers, are based on the wrong text..." He adds, "The first in the long line of manuscripts that were copied for nearly fifteen centuries until the invention of printing... was copied over and over again by scribes who accidentally and even intentionally changed the texts many times." He demonstrates that we do not have the originals [of scriptures] and that we do not even have the first copies of them and in most instances the ones we do have are copies made centuries later. These copies made much later, are strewn with differences between one another. There are "more differences among these manuscripts than there are words in the NT" (sic) itself.

His conclusion is that "the Bible [appears]... as... a human book from beginning to end... was written by different human authors at different times and different places to address different needs." "If god did not perform the miracle of preserving his original words, there is no reason to believe that he performed the miracle of inspiring them in the first place. It should not have been more difficult for god to preserve the words of scriptures than it was to inspire them ..."

Therefore, most importantly, we cannot consider the Bible as a direct line of communication with god. What scriptures tell us is to be accepted on faith alone. One must not forget that the Bible is the only source of what a man called Jesus, who may or may not have existed, is supposed to have said. This is what prompted Stephen J. Gould (renowned Paleontologist) to write, "I would rather peruse 300 pages of Darwin on worms (that he studied) than slog through 30 pages of eternal verities explicitly preached by many writers."

Quoting a non-accredited reference

Christians frequently if not always repeat like trained parrots and in the same mechanistic way such rhetoric as follows without even having thought about what they say:

- The Bible says...
- Jesus said...
- God wants, loves, punishes, pardons and the like.
- Peter said...
- Mark said...
- Luke said...
- Jesus did...
- Noah did...

And the list goes on.

I have just demonstrated that it's not because a book of fiction mentions true cities or places and that it mentions true-life people that the general contents of the book are consequently authenticated, inerrant and true. Though the Bible speaks of certain well-established cities and sites that did and still do exist, and of some true life historical characters Pontius Pilate, Herod), this is not enough to authenticate it as an accurate source for every person or every event that it mentions in its stories.

But, my religious guides tell me that there are dozens of witnesses and often "eyewitnesses" to the events mentioned in scripture; so let's look into the value of their testimony.

CHAPTER 8

EYEWITNESSES THEY SAY

"*[People] who accept [-] testimony at face value [-] are lacking not only in criticism but in the most elementary knowledge of psychology.*"
Carl Gustav Jung, pioneer psychologist

It is time for us to focus on the facts, the data, and overall information, brought by witnesses of key events of the scriptures that would confirm and substantiate them. There are instances where the protagonists of stories in the Bible are either reluctant or incapable of giving their testimony in the events in which they are the actors. One such instance is the story of the adulteress woman and another is Jesus' monologue when he is alone in the garden of Gethsemane. There is no one to witness and record the events: Jesus didn't keep a diary, the adulteress woman wanted to remain anonymous and the disciples were all asleep. Invariably the focus becomes centered on the credibility of the so-called witnesses or authors of scriptures. Let's not forget that many scriptures are nothing more than repetitious liturgies and prayers. The focus on the credibility of the witnesses forces the analysis to become almost archeological and forensic because here, all of these pretended witnesses are now long departed from this world.

Gaius Julius Caesar

Gaius Julius Caesar is a name everyone knows, but how do historians know that he really existed? Just how much of what we have been told of him is true?
Like any important personage, Julius wrote his own accounts of some of his campaigns. We might think that they glorify him in every aspect but they contain very accurate and objective information on the people he confronted. The people he was up against were not keepers of

written records but there were numerous historians at the time who were either Greek or Roman and who corroborated many events and assertions that Caesar made.

Because Caesar was an important person, there were busts made of him, we know what he looked like, and numerous documents attest of many other aspects of his tumultuous life. Some of the more well-known and reliable historians of Caesars era were people like Polybius (202 – 120 B.C.), Posidonius (135 – 51 B.C.), Diodorus Siculus (44 -40 B.C.), Strabo (ca. 64 B.C. - A.D.19), Pliny the Elder (23 – 79 A.D.), Tacitus (ca. A.D. 98), and Athenaeus (ca. A.D. 200), just to name a few.

Not all of these historians wrote about Julius but some of them mentioned events and people that Julius had also described; these writings corroborate his own accounts and confirm their authenticity. Many other historians however wrote about Julius more precisely and there are administrative accounts that give numerous and accurate details about the man; where he was born, of whom he was born, whom he married, who were his children and what he did, where he went and how and when he died and much more. This seems quite logical given that he was a very powerful ruler and because he was for a long time public figure. Therefore, we find it quite normal to have so much information on a person like him. There is no doubt that he really existed and little if any doubt on what he did. If you are interested in learning more about him, there is an incredibly abundant amount of information you can find in libraries and on the internet.

Spartacus

Let us look at another popular figure, Spartacus. His is also a name most people know; Hollywood has made several films relating his life. Here again, how do historians know he really existed?

We have inherited many documents attesting to his reality. We know he was born in Thrace, (Italy), that he escaped from a gladiatorial school in 73 BCE, that he raised an army of about 70,000 slaves and organized a revolt in 72 BCE. The list of things known of him is impressive. We do not have a portrait of him however. Of course, one of the reasons there is so much information known about him is that he caused the ruling administration of the Roman Empire to spend much time and effort in subduing him. His 'exploits' were therefore chronicled carefully.

However, one is somewhat surprised at the amount of chronicled, authenticated and detailed information we know about this man, who never wrote about himself, and who was nothing but a slave and, at first, an obscure gladiator.

- Date of birth: circa 111 BC
- Place of Birth: Area around the middle course of the Strymon (modern-day Struma River, Bulgaria
- Father's name: unknown / Mother's name: unknown
- Date of death:71 BC / Place of death: Battlefield near Petelia (modern-day Strongoli, Calabria, Italy)
- Historians/documents: We have two main sources;
Plutarch of Chaeronea (46-c.122), influential Greek philosopher and author well known for his biographies and his moral treatises is the first. Plutarch informs us that Spartacus was a Thracian from the nomadic tribes. He describes Spartacus' war in his *Life of Crassus*.
Appian of Alexandrea (c.95-c.165) is the second; he tells the same story in his *History of the Civil wars*. Both accounts describe more or less the same events in exactly the same sequence, and it is tempting to see the same source behind their stories, probably the *Histories* of Sallust or (less likely) Livy's *History of Rome from its Foundation*. These two historians give us corroboration and lend credibility to his existence.

Buddha

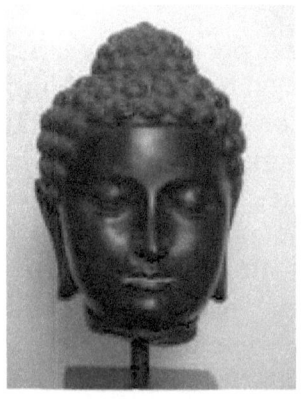

This is not a book on a particular religion. I am just trying to make a point about testimony in historical documents. We will take but a quick blink at this famous figure, Buddha, born in 563 B.C.E. Though there is some uncertainty as to the dates (give or take a few years only), it is well established that what westerners acquiesce as the Buddha, is a man by the name of Siddhartha Gotama (or Gautama). He was a religious philosopher and teacher who lived in India from about 563 to 483 B.C.E. Not one historian would deny his existence, simply because of the abundance of written evidence.

Here we have a figure we know many things about; he was a prince of a province, his mother and father's name are known, they ruled over a people called the Sakyas in northeastern India, etc. We know for example that he too established a lofty and admirable moral philosophy but it is not your usual religion *per se* because he never taught nor pretended to 'divine' incarnation; he is therefore not God, nor his son. Though he was a prince, he gave up his heritage and his comforts and went out into the world to live like the poorest of the poor; this is just to say that if he was in the public eye for some years, he lived most of his life as a humble nobody.

How is it that we know so much about this nobody? He moved people and had many followers; this is not speculated but corroborated, it is attested by many objective written sources. Here is a figure that was born 563 years before the Christian era and yet we have hundreds of documents attesting, corroborating, validating not only the existence of this man but giving ample information on his life and his teachings. This is in stark contrast to the inaccuracies the disinformation and almost inexistent corroborations about an alleged 'Son of God' who lived 563 years later in an era of conquest, of fascinating figures and of numerous and well-versed historians; Jesus the Christ.

Jesus Christ

This brings us to another well-known figure, Jesus the Christ. Just how much do we really know about him? How do historians know he really existed?

The only direct mention a Jesus Christ in written history is that of a Jewish historian, Flavius Josephus, writing for the Roman government in the 70's A.D. (Antiquities of the Jews, Book XVIII, chap. V, p.20; Book XX, chap. IX, p. 140). He confirms that Herod had John the Baptist killed and that he had James, brother of Jesus, who was called 'the Christ', stoned to death. This is however still an item of contention among historians today.

Josephus was born about 37 A.D. and was a Pharisee. Using serious methods, most scholars assume a date of birth for Jesus between 6 and 4 BC, and that Jesus' preaching began around AD 27–29 and lasted one to three years. They calculate the death of Jesus as having taken place between AD 30 and AD 36. This means that Josephus was born about 4 years after Jesus died (in the year 33 AD-average). If Jesus died in 36 AD, Josephus was born in (36 + 4) 40 AD. He would have been 33 when he wrote the text in 70 A.D. which corresponds to (36-Death of Jesus + 33 Age of Josephus) 69 to 70 years after the death of Jesus. Thus, here is a man who could have met followers of Jesus who were in their thirties at the time of the death of Jesus and who would have been at least in their nineties (30 age of witnesses + 60 years after the death of Jesus) when Josephus was in his late twenties. But, from what we know of the average life span of the times, there is very little probability that any eye witness was still alive then.

He wrote a substantial compendium on *The War of the Jews* but, there is in all of this, no more than a fleeting mention of a Jesus. If his text is accurate and reliable, it remains that he is not just talking about an ordinary *fait diver*, a mundane street fight but the death of the 'Son of God'. Is this all that Jesus meant to people at the time, even his own countrymen? Is this all the information this contemporary historian could whip up about what the Gospels acclaim as one of the most transcending persons of his time? But what about the dozens of other noted historians of the times, why do they stay silent?

If it is true that few modern historians would disagree that a man named Jesus truly lived between 4 B.C.E. and about 33 A.D., and that this man gave birth to a lofty ethic and an inspiring ideal of human brotherhood, it still remains troubling that only about 12 direct witnesses carried his message on to other generations. It is extremely troubling that no other more important, independent and objective historians mention him anywhere.

We have no description of him. We do not know where he was really born; some say Nazareth (Mark 6:1) like the Roman sign on his cross was supposed to have said, 'Jesus of Nazareth, King of the Jews' or 'INRI' for short, in Latin; some say Bethlehem (Luke 2:1-7, New International Version). We do not know exactly when he was born. We have no historical confirmation that his mother's name was truly Mary, or that his adopted father was Joseph. People speak of him as Jesus Christ, but without realizing that his last name was not Christ. His mother was not Mary Christ and his father was not Joseph Christ; Christ is a title. Furthermore, could Jesus not write his own diary, biography or precepts? We have no way of knowing any of this.

Whether or not theologians can explain these discrepancies or not, this is not what one would expect, given the accounts of the religious Christian establishment about his miracles, his resurrection and his extraordinary life. Yes, his message is lofty, humbling, and admirable. Yes, he must have taught an appealing philosophy of compassion, justice and equality, but the historical records are particularly disappointing when compared to someone like Spartacus, a mere slave, who managed to unite up to 120,000 slaves and threaten Rome itself.

Here we have been taught that Jesus spoke to hundreds of people, if not thousands, performed incredible miracles, which even today would hit the headlines, and yet no one writes about them during his lifetime. After all the masses that supposedly followed him and after all the supernatural events that he was reputed responsible for or that took place just after his death, no one, not even the Roman historians, think it relevant to mention him in their administrative archives. This is not what one would expect of a man, let alone a son of god, that had such a large influence on his fellow citizens. The true miracle here is the sheer lack of historically corroborated information that surrounds a man that humanity bases its calendar on. The amount of 'disinformation' and legend about this man is appalling.

In conclusion, we only have the Bible (New Testament) to rely upon for basically any information on this Jesus, and therefore the question is can we trust it to be telling the truth, all of the truth and nothing but the truth? The fact that practically no major historians living at the time of Jesus' supposed campaign wrote anything about him does not of course discredit Biblical scriptures, but it fathers doubt and sets the stage for a more in-depth analysis.

Here is a man who lived at a time of numerous other figures many of whom were insignificant in comparison with what Jesus purportedly was, and yet no one writes about him except some of his followers. Yes, his followers write enthusiastically about his teachings, though they sometimes contradict each other; Luke and Mark dispute the birthplace of Jesus; one says it is Bethlehem, the other Nazareth. There are too many contradictions in these writings to list them all here. Just how reliable and accurate are their writings and why were they made so late after his death? Are there not some Homeric embellishments? After all those who wrote about Jesus were biased followers and did not write until long after his death (70 to 100 years) to chronicle his teachings. The fundamental question that should be (or should have been) asked in the first place is "Is the Bible a reliable and therefore authentic and authoritative source of information on Jesus, Yahweh, and whatever godly devices and entities one might see in it"? Unfortunately, the answer to this question, as we are discovering so far, is undeniably NO.

Just who are these people who wrote the scriptures of the Old and New Testaments? There are gospels that have no specified authors such as Genesis, Exodus, Chronicles, Corinthians, Romans and many more. Then there are the Mark, Luke, Matthew, John, James and more. Just what do we know, however, of these presumed authors? Luke for example, has no mother, father, and date of birth we can refer to. Nor do we know where he was born (for sure) or what is his exact relationship to Jesus he speaks of. How many people named Luke were there in the Holy land at the time of Jesus; probably thousands, just like there are thousands of Johns in today's cities and towns? The same can be said of every other presumed author of the other parts of Scriptures attributed to a specific person. This does not exactly clarify the scriptures authenticity at all. The question remains as to the credentials and the basic identity of the authors themselves. It has been often remarked that among the 12 apostles, not many knew how to read let alone write (Acts 4:13; "they were men unlettered"). But more importantly none were reported to take notes and to write a diary.

Objective analysis of the Resurrection

One of the most important passages of the New Testament is the report of the resurrection of Jesus. It is a key element of Christian dogma. Surely this essential part of God's miracle was related by reliable sources with the utmost detail and precision and the witnesses are without a doubt credible. Let us take a close look.

Four gospels report that the tomb of Jesus was found empty by one to an unspecified number of women, one of which would have been Mary Magdalene. There is no precise mention of the purpose of their visit to the tomb, or of the weather (lightning, storm, hot sun?). The time the women visited the tomb varies as well as the number and identity of the women. We have no indication of how many guards there were or who they were (Roman, Jewish, etc.). What could have happened and at what time of day is anybody's guess. We have no description of the messenger(s) they met there (angelic or human). We don't have a detailed rendering of the message they may have received.

Consequently, let us do a forensic approach through six possible scenarios that all have the same credibility using the same amount of information (or lack thereof) than the scriptures offer.

- First scenario; Christ opened the stone "door" with supernatural powers and left without being seen. The guards were asleep or gone, incompetent or bribed; Matthew's Gospel speaks of a bribe seen from the "Christian" point of view.
- Second scenario; grave robbers opened the tombstone and took the body away while the guards slept, were away, or were bribed to turn a blind eye.
- Third scenario; followers of Christ robbed the tomb in the same conditions as in scenario 2 but for different reasons.
- Fourth scenario; Christ opened the tomb and appeared to the guards who were so frightened that they ran away while Christ, who may not have been really dead, escaped.

- Fifth scenario; followers of Christ robbed the tomb and discovered that he was not really dead and healed him back to health.
- Sixth scenario; the women who came to anoint his body found him alive and healed him back to health. The guards had opened the tomb and verified that the body was still there; they concluded that he was indeed dead and left, leaving the tomb opened knowing that someone would come to anoint the body.

There is no need to continue the possibilities. The point is we have no corroborating account, no corroborating evidence from a Roman, another Jewish objective observer such as a Pharisee, a Greek historian, etc. Only one of the scriptural accounts can be truthful but there is the possibility that none of the four accounts is truthful. One thing is certain, they are inaccurate and incomplete. Because of the lack of detailed observations, it appears quite probable that each account is the result of hearsay; the author writes what he heard from someone who heard it from yet someone else. In short, there is no eyewitness. As a matter of fact, there is nowhere to be found, in the entire Bible, the slightest evidence of an eye witness in any of the events concerning Jesus in particular. We are dealing, at best, with hearsay beyond a doubt.

Another consequence of this is the fact that people who claim to have heard God, spoken to God or have received revelations or inspirations from God are unacceptable witnesses to events that cannot be proven. To quote Carl Sagan; "Claims that cannot be tested, assertions immune to disproof are veridically (sic) worthless, whatever value they may have in inspiring us or in exciting our sense of wonder. What they ask you to do comes down to believing, in the absence of evidence on [...] hearsay." Such assertions are those of people who claim having been abducted and having spoken to aliens. Witnessing should always be subjected to verification and corroboration.

What religion asks us to believe of Jesus is truly a huge leap of faith considering the absence of admissible evidence and admissible witnesses and the absence of original scriptural texts. Even if Jesus' birth certificate were to be found tomorrow, this would not prove that what has been said or written about him is true; this is still to be considered as hearsay and certainly not valid, admissible evidence of any sort. One must make the distinction between the existence of a man called Jesus the Christ and the questionable validity of scriptures.

We have also seen, in the case of Mormonism, a perfect example of authentication of scriptures, or miracles or divine whatever, by the simple acceptance of statements made by a handful of persons, witnesses, whose evidence is not admissible in any modern and objective court of law. This is like allowing accusations of witchcraft, made by a couple of irresponsible and foolish teenagers in old Salem, to be received as evidence against innocent people. Nothing in the Bible can be considered admissible in court as evidence because it is all hearsay, myth or legend, but the epitome of irony is that we use it to assure we get in court, the truth, nothing but the truth, from anyone who swears by it. From what we have learned, you can no longer attempt to prove the scriptural truth of the Bible by quoting its self-proclaimed authority. The Bible (and any other scriptural book/s) is not true simply because it says so; this is a circular argument that is not viable.

Now that we know that scriptures are not reliable and sufficient to corroborate the claims of religion, we must turn to another source or argument. My religious guides have been very patient with me and what they have discovered. They hold fast to perhaps a last hope of convincing me; they say that, "We now have to consider and analyze the unavoidable, sacrosanct and convincing arguments for and from miracles".

CHAPTER 9

YOUR FRIEND DOES MIRACLES

What is a miracle?

Richard L. Purtill (1931 – today) professor of philosophy at Western Washington State University wrote, "One traditional way of providing a rational basis for religious belief begins with arguments for the existence of God and [goes on to argue] that a certain body of religious beliefs can be known to be a revelation from God because miracles have been worked in support of those beliefs." His definition of a miracle is; "By miracle we will mean an exception to the natural order of things… caused by the power of God." [In other words, there is no miracle without intervention of God]. For the Biblical writers, miracles signify an "extraordinary coincidence of a beneficial nature" (R.H. Fuller 1996, London).

David Hume (1711-1776) [16], Scottish philosopher, historian, economist, and essayist would add, "But to be a miracle the violation of a natural law would have to be the work of a god who is not a material object. What kind of evidence would we have to have to believe that a divine being had intervened in our world?" He goes on to write, "For there is not to be found, in all history, any miracle attested by a sufficient number of men, of such unquestioned good-sense, education, and learning, as to secure us against all delusion in themselves; of such undoubted integrity, as to place them beyond all suspicion of any design to deceive others; of such credit and reputation in the eyes of mankind, as to have a great deal to lose in case of their being detected in any falsehood; and at the same time, attesting facts performed in such a public manner and in so celebrated a part of the world, as to render the detection unavoidable; all which circumstances are requisite to give us a full assurance in the testimony of men." Hume's justified conditions, though demanding and stringent, are not met by the witnesses of miracles, and of the texts of the Bible in general, and therefore they cannot be considered trustworthy.

R.L. Purtill successfully argues that a miracle could be an exception (violation) of a yet unknown (undetermined) natural law. Today all agree that it is possible (not probable; it is not predictable) for a miracle caused by (a) god to exist, if such a god exists. It could also be that such events have an altogether unknown other cause. But in any case, every scientist and philosopher agrees that miracles are extremely rare in human history and quasi non-existent. This indicates that if this god of miracles exists (take your pick), his presence in human history is extremely rare and quasi inexistent as well. Purtill goes on to state that God uses miracles to reveal to Man a certain body of information. God authenticates (certifies, validates) the words and works of Christ through miracles and in particular the Resurrection; this is authority on the evidence of miracles.

There is only one thing wrong with his argument of authority and authentication. For Christ to perform miracles (including prophesies) he must be God (or at least a lesser god) since by definition a miracle is an act of God. To say that Christ is authenticated by God is to say that Christ (being the incarnation of God) is authenticated by himself. This is a circular argument; God is God because He says so. In other words, God authenticates himself through miracles he creates to authenticate himself (though no one has yet proven that God exists to begin with). This is obviously an absurdity.

Purtill's fantastic criterion

As if it were not enough that miracles are extremely rare events, Purtill goes on to set up limiting criteria. They must not contain "strong" elements of the fantastic, and they must not read like legend, myth or fairy tales. He knows that all other religions have stories that may not be called "miracles" but that have the characteristics of one; such stories have been mentioned around the figure of Buddha for example. Now the stories around Buddha were not called miracles simply because they occurred 600 years before Christ and the term was not in the Buddhist vocabulary, but miraculous events could have occurred. Miracles are said to have occurred with Muhammad and Jewish prophets. If all miracles are to be admitted as possible and valid, then all religions that proclaim miracles are validated; once you have opened the door to admitting miracles, you must accept them all. So, there are rival miracles.

Purtill's attempts at validating Christian miracles by arbitrarily eliminating other religious claims to miracles under the puerile guise of fantasy, is ludicrous and unfounded. He makes a pitiful attempt at discrediting other religion's miracles while attempting to make Christian miracles look plausible with weak arguments. He writes off the miracle of Muhammad riding his horse to the moon as a sheer fantasy but turns right around and declares the Resurrection of Christ as a more reliable and acceptable miracle on just as arbitrary criteria.

However, we all know today of mirages that can be explained by Science. A man of the Bronze-Age watching someone ride off on a horse towards a large rising moon in the desert while a mirage is appearing on the horizon, would likely think that this horseman is riding to the moon. How would this man, ignorant of scientific explanations of mirages, tell the story of what he just saw? Quite obviously he would make it sound like a fantasy and yet he may be perfectly sincere though incapable of giving an objective explanation of his experience. But Purtill's criterion relegates this account to the trash bin and not to the acceptable file of miracle "because it contains strong elements of the fantastic".

This brings up a serious question; why did Christ (God) keep his resurrection such a hush-hush affair when his intention (if we believe religious dogma) is to manifest/authenticate his desire to offer salvation to all of mankind? It appears as if Christ is willing to bring Salvation to his friends only or at most to the "chosen people" of god. Why is this resurrection such a secret, an uncorroborated singularly fantastic account as seen from a skeptic and even scientific point of view (See Chapter 8)? Why didn't Christ simply walk into the grand temple or even Pilate's court yard after his resurrection? What could Christ possibly fear from this demonstration of his miraculous resurrection if at any second he would be "beamed up" by his heavenly father/alter ego? Here again, whether or not the story is woven into a larger context (Salvation, Redemption) of the religion, that could have been invented 70 years after the fact, this miracle is no less fantastic and fairy tale like than one of any other religion.

Benefits from miracles

Religion claims that when a miracle happens to someone, it is widely understood Biblically, that it conveys a benefit to the recipient of this miracle. When considering the account of the Exodus, a giant wave or an opening in a sea that saves the Israelites, religion says Hurrah! After all they are God's people. However, the Egyptians are drowned: Hurrah, again! They are the evildoers, or at least the ones the Judeo-Christian god dislikes. Nevertheless, what have these Egyptians done that is so evil that even god takes part in their demise? We only have the Hebrews side of the story.

With this type of reasoning (sinners vs saints) and this type of punishment for wrongdoing and blessings for good doing, (very subjective issue), we find ourselves faced with the question of the reason for such things as the Holocaust. Was it a punishment from god? Why did He not make a miracle then? Is it harder to open the doors to a concentration camp than it is to open a sea? With this type of reasoning the absurdities and quagmires, abound.

Simon Blackbourn writes in his book *Think*; "Miracles are the kind of thing that, either never happen, or almost never happen; people elevating themselves in the air, lead floating, water turning into wine, the dead coming back to life, someone walking on water, or feed 5000 people with only a few loaves and fishes."

Rewards from a biased god

If a miracle is an act of God, it implies a purpose. It also implies a choice, made by this god. We can only speculate the purpose: punishment, rescue, assistance, healing, revenge, mercy, murder, obliteration, bias, etc.

A sense of implicit benefit to a recipient often accompanies the phenomenon of miracle. When I say a miracle is beneficial to the recipient, it depends on what side of the fence one is on or, might I say, god is on. If miracles were the rewards dispensed by a merciful, just, fair, loving and compassionate god(s), we would finally see thousands if not millions of poor innocent souls eating to fulfillment, curing from horrifically painful diseases and being saved from horrific natural catastrophes such as Tsunamis. Simon Blackbourn (*Think*; 1999) sums this up nicely by saying; "A little miracle or two snuffing out the Hitlers and Stalins would seem far more useful than one that changes water to wine."

Miracles are not only insufficient to authenticate the feedback (accessibility) of god(s), but, as David Hume would say, "Since almost all religions attest to miracles, they must all be true. But how can this be?" Once again, even if miracles were receivable evidence for feedback (accessibility) from god, they would ironically validate several religions all at once.

The simpler the better

I have put emphasis on the plethora of needless religious extravaganzas and accounts that religion presents in an attempt to justify or authenticate principles and dogma that could easily be explained with much less fanfare. William of Ockham (1288-1348, England) devised a simplistic but efficacious principle called Ockham's razor which states that where there is a choice between two theories (or scenarios) the simplest is more likely to be correct [and I would add the most intelligent, and useful].

The point here is that a god whose principal attributes (according to scripture) are omnipotence and omniscience should in, all logic, be able to edify a plan of action that would be as simple and as efficacious as possible. But, as we have seen through the previous chapters and analyses, He loves to complicate matters to the absurd.

We have discovered that there is much doubt as to the origin of Judeo-Christian-Islamic scriptures. They are not corroborated by other objective texts of history, they are not what an omniscient god would be expected to dictate or inspire and they are mingled with myth, legend and errors of all sorts. We are left wondering if religions have had contact or any communication of any sort with their god. What other forms of contact or communication are there left? Is there anyone still out there that really knows who this invisible friend is?

===========================

Here is a possible example of a kind of miracle without any particular, evident purpose; a three-million-year-old extinct shell with two species of equally extinct corals growing on it. What are the odds of such an association and what are the odds that after 2.6 Million years in the ground it would be found in one piece? Think about it.

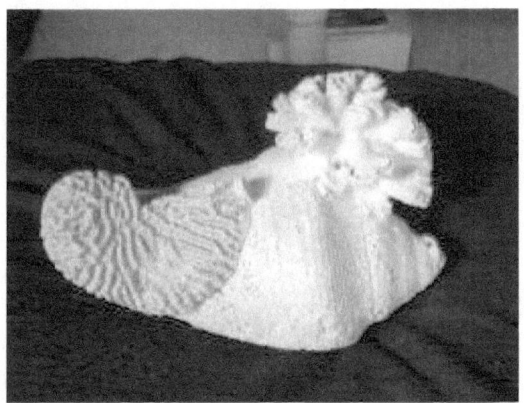

CHAPTER 10

SO, WHO KNOWS GOD?

"The prestige of the obscure in the view of children and the simple minded is certain."

Maurice Barrès (French author)

Let us summarize what we have discovered.

- Prayer, sacrifice and divine revelation or inspiration is not an efficacious or unequivocal means of communicating with a god.
- The scriptures have not been corroborated and can't be.
- This god is the epitome of ambiguity:
    1. He is loving, yet abusive.
    2. He is not all loving (He has conditions to his love) because He loves those who follow Him more than those who do not.
    3. Generous but, demanding all in retribution
    4. Good yet evil; He is not merciful and benevolent because He allows sufferance of innocents.
    5. He is biased, takes sides in conflicts, games, and even storms.
    6. Capable of creating storms or floods to destroy his enemies but incapable of stopping one from killing innocent women, children and even priests, or the destruction of a Church during an earthquake, a fire, etc.
    7. He is said to be intelligent, but his creation has no apparent purpose and makes no rational sense unless seen through the theory of evolution; example, predation.
    8. He sent us text messages that are incoherent and far from what one would expect the greatest mind to be capable of.
    9. Most importantly, He is incapable of sending us in today's highly technical environment the slightest E-mail or phone

call to assure us of His well-being or of his good-intentions or just a Christmas card.
And the list goes on.

Yet from the abyss of His infinite universe He finds time, so religion claims, to tinker and toy daily with minute particles of dust to assure the happiness of each particle. How can there be so little evidence for God and yet so many people who pretend to know Him? The Roman Catholic Church teaches the doctrine of papal infallibility. In other words, the Pope speaks for Jesus and thus God. This of course has been a subject of contention since the Reformation and the cause of the schism with the Protestant Church. It is contentious to this day. The only other official Church to pretend that its leader(s) speaks directly for God and to God is the Mormon Church. Here is an official statement by the official Church of LDS "As members of The Church of Jesus Christ of Latter-day Saints, we are blessed to be led by living prophets—inspired men *called to speak for the Lord*, as did Moses, Isaiah, Peter, Paul, Nephi, Mormon, and other prophets of the scriptures. We sustain the President of the Church as *prophet, seer,* and *revelator—the only person on the earth who receives revelation to guide the entire Church*. We also sustain the counselors in the First Presidency and the members of the Quorum of the Twelve Apostles as *prophets, seers, and revelators.* [17]

The '*Knowers*' of god

I have received from well-intentioned people the classic "God bless you" (without having sneezed) and have responded by an appreciative thank you. But as an atheist I consider this superfluous though I can understand that in some circumstances certain people just blurt it out without a second thought. Could it be that these people, by assuring me that I will be blessed, have the supernatural power to intercede for me? Do these well-intentioned people have the power to really speak to god (for me or themselves) and know what He wants and says? Which god, which religion is the one that is going to bless me? Which one are they praying to and what is their place in the intercession? Who are these people who can communicate with this god so easily?
Ever since the beginning of his life in social groups Man has invented gods in an attempt to explain away events in his life such as rain,

storms, animals, volcanoes, stars and hundreds of other natural and seemingly unnatural (not to say, supernatural) phenomena he has been the witness of. We cannot blame our ancestors for this because they had no way, no tools, to interpret what they witnessed. Their conception of the world was based on their perceptions, their senses, their fears, their anxieties in other words on their feelings and illusions and irrationalities.

When certain patterns reoccurred now and then, like phases of the moon, their interpretations were often sound and correct. But when their interpretations were based solely on their phantasms and what they thought they experienced, their conceptions were often outrageous by our standpoints. They had no other reference points, no standards to compare them to. This explains the pure invention of hundreds of gods of the most imaginative forms and powers. History shows an almost unbelievable menagerie of gods of all sorts: animal gods, half animal-half human gods and then gods in human form.

The epitome of this evolution came when they entrusted their fears and anxieties to people who pretended to have, or were believed to have special powers and especially the power to access god(s), to speak to god(s). These people were given special privileges and powers because they were not only revered but also feared. Some even became gods or sons/daughters of gods (Pharos, Kings, Queens, etc.). They all soon learned that their privileges would assure them prestige, comfort, wealth, and a life of luxury and leisure. They soon learned that by grouping their efforts and institutionalizing their "shows", authoritative rules, codes and philosophies they would assure their positions for life.

These institutions that we still call today religions, churches and denominations, became the first enslavement of generations of human minds. They imposed a blind acceptance of something not supported by reason, simply by the authority of their (personal) source. In other words, these privileged people imposed religion on the premise that they alone had access to god(s), sometimes to the consequence of torture and death, which they often happily and diligently carried out themselves. Just think of the millions of people who have worshiped, knelt down to, died for, killed for, grotesque gods of all sorts and all this in the name of their god and cheered on by these '*knowers*' of god. How disgusting and insane this would seem to highly advanced and intelligent aliens visiting our planet if none of these gods is real and if all of the people who pretended to know them were frauds.

Even if there was a divine essence, a god or even several gods that exist independently of human conceptions, He would exist in such a way that we are incapable of imagining, of conceiving, of detecting his very nature. Ironically by making this god so outrageously inaccessible, "We can never know and define any aspect of this essence. Indeed, any conception of the divine essence made by Man can only be illusionary and irrationally based. Whatever concept we may come up with can only be a vague approximation at best and most probably a mistake all together. Theism bases its god on unsubstantiated illusions made only of words". [Don Cupitt, 1990][18] I have to say that this quote is taken out of context but ironically it fits the situation quite nicely.

Irrelevance

Let us forget playing the organ at mass some religionists say today. Let's play the guitar, let's bring in a rock group. Let's forget the Latin Vulgate, no longer understood, and pray in English or whatever other language you speak. Let's forget the Sabbath, eat meat on Friday, and abandon the Saints (Protestantism). Let's not slaughter our neighbors who don't obey to the Pope, let's not impale them, nor stone them, nor roast them alive, but let's just have a pig/lamb roast and an old fashion shindig instead. What matters after all is that we show and apply that good old loving feeling. Let's keep silent about the times when we applauded god's vengeance. Let's forget that people have been told to address themselves to god(s), in Hebrew, then in Aramaic, then in Greek, then in Latin, and even in only one particular language and then recently in any other language they want. So, what will it be? One can only wonder if religion, after killing millions of people for what now appear to be ridiculous offenses, just doesn't reinvent its dogmas as society evolves.

There seems to be a tendency, today, to consider church as a place to get together, sing songs, have an experience and love one another in accordance with "Christ's-Calling". Some Christians even think that Jesus didn't care whether people were gay. But the Bible is clear, homosexuality is a sin. People were excommunicated for breaking much lesser rules and the cities of Sodom and Gomorrah were destroyed for nuances of this type. These two cities have been used as metaphors for vice and homosexuality. The English word *sodomy* derives from this story and is used particularly in homosexual references. Islamic punishments are sometimes associated with

Sodom and Gomorrah in sharia law. These two cities are mentioned in the Old Testament (Hebrew Torah) Book of Genesis and in the New Testament, as well as in the Quran and the hadith.

If god(s) exists and he can 'hear' us, and 'see' us and understand any language we speak and if he cares about us, He should listen when one speaks to him. He should listen whether you stand, kneel, stoop, bow, prostrate yourself, hold a candle, a nail, a hammer, a cross, a feather, a pipe, a whistle, a horn, a drum, a stone, a jewel, a sacrifice, an offering, ... whatever; whether you are clothed in silk, in cotton, in polyamide, in tweed, or in nothing at all. The way one 'must pray', the way one 'must act', the way one 'must dress', according to any one of the Knowers of god mentioned above, is irrelevant, as irrelevant as your first shirt or even your first diaper when it comes to your relationship to God.

Consequently, what do religions know that many of us presumably do not? We have discovered that religions have no evidence that they have a unique access to God, any god. So what gives them the right to claim truth if they have no authority, authenticity or validity? ... Nothing! If God exists, no human being can possibly know or even imagine what God is. Therefore, your interpretation of God is as good as anybody else's, even that of so-called priests, pastors, shamans, rabbis, bishops, popes and the like. In this perspective, we are all knowers of God and what we all know is nothing.

Why do we need a god?

When I questioned those who could see their invisible friend, my question was often why I needed this invisible friend in the first place, to the risk of appearing facetious. I usually got the same litany of the following category of answers with varied degrees of consistency and/or vehemence, and not always in this order:
- You need him because he loves you and wants to help you.
- You need him because you have sinned and must save your soul.
- Because he can heal you and give you the wonderful life he has planned for you.
- He is the only way to heaven.
- He is the only way to avoid hell.

There are many more but they all boil down to these essential five answers. A short dialogue on why we need God too often sounds like this; "We need him to protect us". Atheist: "Against what?" Religionist: "To save us from ourselves and from our original sin." Ah, of course the original sin, another myth.

Retrospectively, and according to scriptural texts, this god creates an imperfect being (Man) to whom he dictates commandments or divine laws and expects this imperfect being to obey. Whether or not these divine laws are just or not, is irrelevant because Man is imperfect and when tempted, will inevitably breach the laws. As soon as man breaches the laws this god calls it a sin. Thus, this god by imposing divine laws He knows will be breached, He invents Sin intentionally. Besides, we are told that He has the plan all along to send his son to absolve the sins. But, why would a God all-loving and all-merciful, create an imperfect being only to submit him to laws that he cannot abide by?

Without a god

On the other hand, the absence of god brings us to an interesting consequence. If God does not exist, then there are no divine laws to breach and therefore no sin if we understand sin as a breach of the divine laws. Consequently, we cannot say that we need God to pardon our sins because without him there are none. This is one of the bases for my change of paradigm.

Another reason put forth by religionists, for the necessity of a god is that without one we would have nothing but cold technology and emotionless science to guide our moral compass, and that could not possibly work. Frankly, why does a 5-year-old child have an innate sense of justice and fairness while a 50-year-old needs a supernatural invisible-Cop to tell him/her how to behave? If you don't understand what compassion, empathy, justice, equality, fraternity, altruism, liberty, indiscrimination, love, etc., is, by the age of 18 then you need either psychiatric help or some complimentary re-education.

How can any of the tyrannical, misogynistic, abusive, and Bronze-age Father-deities possibly be of any help with stories of myths and legends? Deities declared to be all-powerful and all-knowledgeable but who cannot just send us a phone call and to whom one has to pray as if this supernatural telepathic method is more efficacious than modern technology.

Are these gods computer and phone illiterate and technically challenged? To answer this question properly, it would likely take serious and objective studies or surveys to refer to, but I don't know of any recent ones.

Humanity's premise has always been that we exist because of an eternal something, yet unknown or inaccessible, when in reality this eternal something exists only because we do; it is the creation of our own psyche. Ask a tree, a lion, a giraffe if there is an eternal something. The world needs us to exist; without any intelligent being to contemplate it, there would be no world.

Why young adults abandon religion

One is generally drawn into religion by one's parents or one's social environment. Every individual should be allowed to discover and cultivate his/her relationship with a higher entity (god if you wish) or just spirituality through a personal quest and without outside pressure of any sort. We all have the duty to learn, to study, to accumulate information, knowledge, and therefore to enrich our "software of life".

Religion has a creed, a set of principles and rules, rites, codes. They are immutable. These seemingly innocuous, little details are the very reasons why people were impaled, raped, tortured, burned, crucified, slaughtered with the utmost finesse and refinement that would make even a Satan cry. When young educated adults reflect on this history, they inquire about these little differences that make what religion is all about. They think twice about turning a blind eye to these minor details that people have died for and wonder if simple Belief (personal and unique), simple compassion, simple Humanism is not better than institutions.

Whatever the reasons for the undeniable trend to shy away from religion, it most certainly has to do with this information revolution. Computers allow for inquiry and an objective (if not only subjective at first) but discrete and stealth personal quest. Despite the peer pressure and even "parental controls", any young inquisitive adult can ask questions about religion, about dogma, religious history and even explore beyond a religion, the domains of agnosticism and atheism if they dare. What is more, they can debate and discuss the subjects with people they don't know and who don't know them, giving them more courage and freedom to explore any topic, or aspect of a topic they wish, without the fear of ostracism: This is the advantage of the domain of the "Blog", or as some call it, the "Blogosphere".

No more inhibitions, no more inquisitive looks, no more taboos or hesitations to ask what used to be forbidden questions, no more forbidding walls. There is no more excuse then for a young adult to be ignorant of simple questions about religion and no excuse to not have at least a personal, logical answer. I personally have faith in the intelligence and open-mindedness of today's youth.

The Guilt-forever-syndrome

I have watched many hours of televangelists and been to many sermons in various places. What did I get out of it? If I set aside the boring rhetorical quotes from the Bible and the litany of interpretations made to make me feel guilty, unworthy and in need of something else but my lowly life and self, it's the understanding that religion preys on fear.

Religion has perfected what I call the Guilt-forever-syndrome; a very efficacious self-regenerating psychosis. It works like this; I can't see my invisible friend which is my first infirmity. So, because of this visual impairment, I need to work on believing he exists but, why? For a plethora of reasons, the first of which is that I am a sinner, for no fault of my own but, originating from a fault of some imaginary first human called Adam. It just so happens that this invisible "friend" wants to punish *ad infinitum* all of Adam's "descendants" because the booboo that he committed was really a big one and it really upset this invisible friend to a point that I can't even imagine.

Here comes the intricacy of this scheme; this invisible friend sent his son to die for Adams sins but I must not commit new ones or else. Thus I must spend the rest of my life working hard to be a good girl or boy; that includes going to and giving to the church. This also entails wondering, day in and day out, how I must best act. From this ensues constantly repenting for what I perceive as possible infractions, at the drop of a pin, thus constantly worrying and asking myself if such and such little unlucky event is not a sign of my treason. This is how people get caught up in this cycle of guilt, repentance, new guilt, new repentance… forever and ever. It is the equivalent of the Minotaur's maze, a veritable web of subtle but deadly traps that keep the believer turning incessantly in circles while religion watches from the center of the maze and rejoices at its ruse.

It is the epitome of irony that for thousands of years, religion has been seen as the Temple of human thought, when all the while it has been the Pinnacle of nonsensical thinking.

CHAPTER 11

DEATH OF THE MINOTAUR

We have seen that scriptures are not reliable sources of information on pretty much anything concerning God. What is more, the typical attributes of God as given by religious texts (Bible) only confound the problem, remember;

- He is immaterial (John 4:23-24)
- He is invisible (Genesis 32:22-30; Exodus 24:9-11; 1 Timothy 1:17; Deuteronomy 4:15; Job 9:11; Matthew 6:6; Romans 1:20; Colossians 1:15; Hebrews; 11:27; 1 John 4:12)
- He is undetectable (Job 11:7-8 & 26:14 & 37:23; Psalms 145:3; Isaiah 40:28; 55:8-9; 1 Timothy 6:16)
- He is eternal (Psalm 102:25-27; Hebrews 1:10-12; 13:8)
- He is omniscient (Psalm 139:2-6; Isaiah 40:13-14)
- He is omnipotent (Genesis 18:14; Luke 18:27; Revelation 19:6)
- He is ubiquitous (Psalm 139:7-12)

See no god, hear no god ...

We are confronted with two possibilities. First of all, if a god communicates through natural means, He/She/It can theoretically and inevitably be detected and thus scientifically revealed. Unfortunately, these communications have never been recorded or corroborated. Because God is immaterial, He is not visible, measurable or detectable in any way; He is not a force or magnetic or atomic manifestation. He is quite mysterious since no one can see Him, smell Him, hear Him, touch Him, or taste Him. Consequently, until God, or this divine essence, decides to reveal itself to us in an unequivocal manner by some sort of direct intervention stripped of the slightest ambiguity, we have no right to deduce or conclude that He is a male entity, that his name is Smith, that he has a beard, that he gave us a son, or a daughter, or that we are in his image or that He has eight arms, a crown, a white robe or any other such attire. All this is unsubstantiated irrationality. Secondly, let us consider the possibility that a god (or several gods) exists but that He is of another dimension or scale, then He can only remain a sheer mystery. He, or any other such god, is totally inaccessible. The impossibility of ever communicating would be such that we would have no hope of ever knowing this god. Therefore, if this god, or any other, resides in a supernatural domain and communicates essentially, if not strictly, through supernatural agencies, there is no hope of scientific evidence. This also means that, unless one has supernatural powers, no one can communicate with something that can only be accessed by supernatural forces.

A quick review of the essential attributes of God, according to scriptures shows that Religion has paradoxically constructed a god that is so extreme He has become inaccessible even to religion itself. Scriptures inevitably appear then as a pitiful stone-age attempt to make God seem accessible while creating a being so inconceivable that it takes supernatural powers to communicate with him. The invention of a Messiah only compounds the paradox by creating a man who is a god and yet who has none of the attributes of a god; mortal (born of woman, and aging), physical (material), limited (having specific dimensions), not omnipotent though capable of a few miracles, in other words not presenting the usual attributes of a god. (See list above).

Yet, we are asked to believe that someone knows the exact name of God, when we do not even have proof that He, She or It exists. Here is our witness, who has never seen the suspect, who says he knows his exact name, because he heard it somewhere, or read in an uncorroborated text, or even dreamed it. It is no wonder that Christians use the presumed likeness of Jesus as an image of God since there is no other. God made Man in his image, so there is some logic in projecting Man's image back to God especially when His son Jesus is supposed to have looked like one of us. But, in the other scriptural religions, god is never represented in image and it is often a heresy to even try. Under these circumstances, any attempt by religion to identify this god would be akin to a description in a criminal investigation of a suspect that has never been seen, for whom there exists, no physical observation, no picture, portrait, for whom the only tangible evidence is to be accepted through simple hearsay, on the basis of witnesses who have long passed away. This would (and should) outrage any respectable judge, jury, court and intelligent person.

The inaccessible god

Religions claim to have the power to supernaturally communicate with their god(s). Science and simple common sense as well as our analysis of prayer and scriptural invalidity prove that there has never been the slightest communication between a God and man. Science may not be able to disprove god, but it disproves any and all claims of communication between God and religion. The bottom line is, if we cannot access god, it is as if he didn't exist: "Can't know god = No god".

Unfortunately for religion, despite thousands of years of prayer, there is to this day absolutely no recorded, objective, substantiated way in which god has responded directly to a prayer. This does not mean that He has not in some 'mysterious' way. But, there is absolutely no way that we can ever know if our messages have ever gotten through because there has never been a substantiated, non-equivocal, scientifically recorded 'feedback'. Many stories abound about such things as miracles but they are all circumstantial, based on hearsay and could never be accepted in a court of law as evidence of anything.

In substance, a one-way communication is the equivalent to no communication at all. There cannot be and will never be any rational way to prove the existence of God (or gods) unless He chooses to reveal Himself. Because there has never been such an event, no one, absolutely no one can say that they have formal proof of the existence of a god. As we have seen, no sacred written document proves the existence of a God either. There is no formal evidence whatsoever.

Let us summarize our findings:
- If god exists and prayers get through to Him, they can only establish a one-way communication unless god responds and establishes an 'access' to Man, but there is to this day no evidence of such a liaison. Because god is inaccessible to Man, prayer is most likely to be an illusion when used as a means of direct communication. Prayer, consequently, can only be seen as a placebo for psychological health and harmony in our irrational needs.
- As defined by religion, miracles and angels are and always have been myths or legends. There is not to this day the slightest

- irrefutable, substantiated and admissible evidence for their existence. There are neither messengers nor messages from God.
- At this point in our technological and historical evolution, god is inaccessible to Man. In addition, there is, to this day, no substantiated, unequivocal and admissible evidence that God has ever 'accessed' Man.
- Until new technology enables Man to have access to God, or until God manifests himself in an unequivocal, substantiated and irrefutable manner, He will remain a mystery.

Maybe God has abandoned us to our foolishness once and for all. It would be no wonder then that god has not sent a message to us in this century of communication satellites, radio and television not to mention computers.

Inaccessism

In conclusion of this passage, God (at least the one of scriptural religion) is undeniably inaccessible to Man and Man is inaccessible to God. This inaccessibility of one to the other abolishes, '*ipso facto*', the authenticity, authority and validity of any and all religions that profess scriptures 'dictated' by (a) god. This is the principle of *inaccessism*.

The consequences of Inaccessism are humbling;

1. Man is not the special creature of a god, any god.
2. Man is not the purpose, nor the center of the universe.
3. Man is sole responsible for his actions.
4. An inaccessible god renders religion obsolete.

The aphorism of this analysis could well be;

"Know communication = know god,
But, "No communication = no god."

Theology, a misnomer

God is not accessible at this stage of our history. Consequently, one cannot pretend to study something that one has no access to or something no one has ever had access to. How then can religion eventually pretend to study this invisible friend? One very serious consequence of inaccessism is that the term Theology (from the Greek Theo = god and Logos = study), or the study of God, becomes absurd and the term is a misnomer; there is no studying God if He is not and never was accessible. Unless theologians have supernatural powers, they cannot study a supernatural being. All that they can study are the scriptures with their historical and social interactions of groups of people, called sects, which had or have a common set of philosophical opinions and doctrines on a given concept of a god or gods: the scriptures are their only access and we know that they are not from God. Theology should be replaced by a new name such as *Sectology*.

Karen Armstrong [19] (British author and commentator) writes in her book, *the Case for God* (2009), page 308, "In the past, theologians have found it useful to have an exchange of views with atheists. But, it is difficult to see how theologians could dialogue fruitfully with [Richard] Dawkins, [Sam] Harris, and [Christopher] Hitchens because their theology is so rudimentary. We should, however, take careful note of what we might call the Dawkins phenomenon. The fact that these intemperate antireligious tracts have won such wide readership not only in secular Europe but in religious America suggests that many people who have little theological training have problems with the *modern God*. Some believers are still able to work creatively with this symbol, but others are obviously not. They get little help from their clergy, who may not have had an advanced theological training and whose worldview may still be bounded by the *modern God*. *Modern theology* is not always easy reading. Theologians should try to present it in an attractive, accessible way to enable congregants to keep up with the latest discussions and the new insights of Biblical scholarship, which rarely reach the pews."

This pompous, biased and irrational rambling about theological training, that has been going on for over two millennia, is supposed to supersede any intellectual philosophy coming from some of the most well-grounded and analytical minds of the $20^{th}/21^{st}$ century. As if these super-theologians could twist their scriptures to better adapt to the public at large, make them more accessible and attractive, more modern and adapted to the insights [read, interpretations of yet previous interpretations, *ad nauseum*] and discussions of our time when they themselves apparently have no idea of what they really mean anyway. How could they? They have no access to a god, any god: The texts they continue to interpret have been written by human beings and have been copied, re-copied, re-edited, tortured, twisted and mingled with innumerable myths and legends, over hundreds of years. These scriptures are so inextricable that no amount of tortuous "advanced theology" could ever make sense of them. They are so mystical that when they say one thing they mean another. The reality of it is that they make no sense at all whatever way anyone tries to understand them. When they say god is omniscient, omnipotent, ubiquitous ... it means that He is, but only in some specific supernatural circumstances that only an "advanced theologian" [read, charlatan] can explain. Even for Pope Francis, the scriptures can be completely re-invented [20]. In October, 2014, he declared, among other things, that "the belief that God created the world in six days and the account in the book of Genesis is an allegory for the way God created the world": So much for a so-called inerrant "Word of God" that was used to torment free-thinkers for centuries.

So, why do we continue to offer titles of PHD in theology to people whose minds gravitate around principles of instant gratification through prayer and sacrifice; graduates who are proponents of gathering people in doctrines and dogmas that isolate them from the real world and keep them in irrational dream worlds? 'Doctors' who are incapable, after all they have studied, of bringing one shred of evidence to their personal ability, or to the ability of any other living person for that matter, to correspond (supernaturally) with God. Nor can they scientifically or rationally demonstrate that God is accessible in any of the ways their doctrines and dogmas pretend. They have no more merit, nor power to access God or spirits than the common medium or crystal ball gazer. This is why I will not indulge in the slightest Bible study or turn to these so-called scriptural scholars for guidance.

Religion, from the standpoint of Inaccessism, appears as a king or emperor divested of his crown and of his symbols of authority, a senile impotent pathetic character in need of serious psychotherapy. Religion is a school of perpetual mental ailments based on the premise that you are ill and must heal from a guilt-forever-syndrome that it breeds in each gullible mind through a permanent and persistent conditioning; somewhat like a hamster in a cage that has a stationary wheel that allows the hamster the illusion of freedom but that can only go in circles. It teaches a subservient attitude towards charlatans who know nothing more than their victim about an invisible eye-in-the-sky, but who have them on a leash and abuse their confidence, their innocence, their vulnerability and who should be helping them to obtain the medical assistance they really need.

A quick look in the hundreds of monotonous, tedious, boring, humdrum, mundane, dreary, tiresome, recurrent, and repetitious publications, incessantly written by Reverends, Bishops, religious and lay persons of every stripe and continually printed by religious schools, colleges and institutes (such as one ironically "for Psychological Sciences"), shows a litany of traps laid out for the sole purpose of capturing the vulnerable victim into the stationary wheel. In one of these that I refuse to recognize because it is not worthy of recognition like most of them, I found in three consecutive pages of about 400 words each, the word healing mentioned 16 times, the word wound, 4 times, the word redemption (redeemed/redemptive), 3 times, the word sin, 4 times, the word suffering, 3 times, the word brokenness, 2 times and the words evil, trauma judgment, and even therapy mentioned one time each, leading to a type of martyr complex. It even has the audacity to cite, "a team of psychologists and neurologists" that it cannot and does not identify but that it uses as a smoke screen to lure the candidate into its non-medically recognized and un-accredited psychology and philosophy of "healing", thus blending a pseudo medical and pseudo-scientific approach to religious doctrine. True, certified, medical psychiatric doctors should be outraged at the idea that religion is prostituting its discipline and offering to those who need real therapy, magic texts, magic potions, magic CDs, DVDs and other paraphernalia to their prospective patients. The scriptures are being presented as a dumbed-down version of a manual of psychiatry that is not only counterfeit but dangerous while the Pope himself is presenting them as a dumbed-down version of a science book that is not only counterfeit but dangerous for the rationality, sanity and education of our young people.

Is the human mind really incapable of simple clarity and understanding? Perhaps deep down inside our psyche there is a "demon" that is needy and avid for sympathy and attention but who also has a martyr complex. Religion jumps on the opportunity to dish out false love and false sympathy in exchange for an everlasting subjugation and servitude to its inaccessible god and its institutions at the cost of ones' rationality and intellectual freedom and even sanity.

Life without god

It may surprise some of you but, if we have been living with a god who is completely inaccessible we have been living in reality without a God. Consequently, those who pretend that we cannot live without a god are wrong because we have been living quite well without one all along.

Life without God has interesting consequences:

- We would no longer see martyrs for an invisible nothing, no more suicide bombers; an inaccessible god kills religion.
- Life is a random happening, a lucky mix of matter and energy.
- There could be no such thing as Heaven or Hell, or Sin (breach of divine law).
- Death is nothingness, oblivion.
- If god does not exist and has never existed, how sad to think of all the energy wasted and the blood spilled by millions of people for an illusion.
- Whether we live morally or not, the end is the same, nothingness.
- How much more valiant and chivalrous to live morally, knowing that the only reward is here and now and not after death, knowing that the only reward is in the recognition and gratitude of our human counterparts and not in some utopia called heaven.
- Our heroes would (hopefully) no longer be generals and conquerors but compassionate, humble and loving everyday *saints* such as scientists who find cures, rescuers who save lives, etc.
- Life could become a much more valuable asset that one would not gamble away or steal away from someone else. By assessing the nullity of a myth called Heaven, we would give value to life. There would no longer be anyone to gamble their only earthly existence on an illusory and subjective heaven, in the name of a lost cause, a futile honor or glory

especially by cheating innocent others out of their own precious lives as well.
- True well-being does not demand belief in the supernatural, but in reason.
- People like me (skeptics, etc.) who can't see an invisible friend are not only part of the norm, they are the norm.

We have come full circle. We as grown adults, (religious guides and readers), have just penetrated the inner sanctum of the maze and we have killed the Minotaur. I finally understand why I could not see this invisible friend nor hear him or speak to him; He is not accessible. I have healed from my impairments that I really didn't have in the first place. I have broken free from the Guilt-forever-syndrome and I hope that you have too. The fear of something that doesn't exist is perhaps the worst type of paranoia and the worst type of subjugation: We will return to this issue in another volume. Religion is like the Minotaur, it lurks in the deepest recesses of the meanderings of our primitive brain; it is like the monster under the bed of your early years, it feeds on your primordial fears and it makes of you a puppet, a zombie to its fantasies. But we have killed the Minotaur and we have come out of the maze; we are free.

We have discovered the misinterpretations and even the mendacity of religions that have no authority and no authenticity but still have a strong hold on gullible souls who need to visualize, see god as a personal friend, a likeness of their own and a key to an illusory heaven. Religion is trying to make a comeback by twisting its scriptures to explain the universe in a way that matches the discoveries of Science and pretending that it knew all along the constitution of the universe, the existence of a big-bang, black holes, and multiverses. This is quite a stretch and a complete distortion of its sacred texts. We have shown that religions have no absolutes only empty recipes that are not based on any reality. For centuries religion used its scriptures as a crystal ball to find insights into the truths of the world. Now religion is locked up inside its crystal ball looking out at a universe beyond its capacity to comprehend and beyond the capacities of its scriptures to explain.

Stop admiring those who continue to pretend that they can see their invisible friend or even speak to him and start feeling sorry for them. We have discovered that we, the skeptics, are not just part of the norm, but that we are the norm. It is time for Medical Science to finally declare religion a mental disorder so that we can intern some of its more acute cases and help them recover. They should be treated like people who claim to have seen aliens and have been abducted. It is time to heal.

CHAPTER 12

A TIME FOR HEALING

Did you say hallucinations?

Richard Dawkins was once asked by an elderly gentleman what he would say to a man who for over 50 years communicated with Jesus on a regular basis. Dawkins answers, "You are obviously sincere but I think that you are hallucinating, that is all I can say." [21] (Not verbatim). Is this response that cruel or simply a diagnosis of sorts made by a man who is a scientist and who sees this behavior as abnormal? This response is brutal but polite. Is there any verity in his conclusion?

All of us who have taken the time to thoroughly analyze religion in this quest have discovered a pernicious aspect of religious belief. It does not suffice to conclude that scriptural religions have no authority, validity or authenticity and that they are based solely on myth, legend and hearsay, it is the cause of and the petri dish of mental disorders that only licensed psychotherapy can remedy. It is my turn to be brutal and direct.

If no one has yet openly dared to envision the whole of religious experience and belief as a psychosis it's because its authenticity and validity have been empirically, authoritatively and implicitly accepted as unquestionable. But, after what we have discovered, the conclusion is inevitable and obvious. I am not a medical doctor and this is not a cheap attempt at defaming religion. I am a scientist and we have seen that religion stifles science by allowing religious patients for example to think that if they cure from cancer or whatever disease… it's a miracle from their god, though they go to the hospital for treatment instead of staying at home in prayer. We are doing science a disfavor by allowing this charade to continue.

To paraphrase Victor Stenger, what can religion bring to science? It brings an otherworldly god beyond our access that is not worth scientific research and who is useless to worship. What can Science bring to religion; psychotherapy.

Seriously, my real contention here is that much of the rituals and teachings of religions cause situational experiences that are prone to provoking forms of anxiety, hallucinatory reactions and more, including a form of specific phobia that should be defined as psychopathology. Psychopathology is a term which refers to either the study of mental illness or mental distress or the manifestation of behaviors and experiences which may be indicative of mental illness or psychological impairment. Psychiatrists and clinical psychologists are particularly involved in clinical treatment of mental illness, or research into the origin, development and manifestations of such states. So why is religion off limits? It appears obvious that it is the perfect breeding ground for such ailments. I understand that it is not the role of modern medical science to point an accusative finger at religion declaring that it is the cause of such disorders, but it could perhaps someday agree officially that believing in an invisible, undetectable, immaterial etc. friend, and pretending to see and speak to Him... is a mental disorder worthy of psychoanalysis and treatment.

One of my guides jumps at the opportunity to throw one of those ritualistic nonsensical phrases. "But, God is not an object of worship but a *presence* dwelling within us, a force surrounding us and a *principle* by which we live." My response is, "As eloquent as this sentence may be, it doesn't mean anything rational or concrete. It is the typical religious mystical mumbo jumbo of all religious charlatanism. A *principle* is a concept not a physical being. Something experienced in you (*presence*) is probably associated with your psyche and therefore in your mind; so what this says is that God is a figment of your imagination. As for the force around you, it is the pressure of the air above you and the electro-magnetic force of gravity. No other relevant force has yet been discovered. In conclusion, your God is not a material thing, He basically does not exist; He is just a concept in your head."

Even though many of us have broken free from the Guilt-forever-syndrome, there lingers on a fear in others, that has been meticulously cultivated, meticulously exploited and meticulously preserved by the church, the priests, and all the associated charlatans so as to continue to harvest time, money, and support from the person or persons so conditioned that they can never truly or easily break loose from religion's grip. We have destroyed the claims that religion knows a god. We have not shown that no god exists but we have shown that we do not need to fear the retributions of a god with who we have never had any communication. So you may still have an invisible fear, but you should no longer have an invisible friend. This invisible fear is also in need of some sort of therapy, but we will consider this in a second volume.

There is some trauma in discovering that what you have believed in most of your life is in fact an illusion. There is also some negation of ailment in the first place; hoarders for example always deny that they are. Non-religious people do not have a visual impairment or a hearing one either, but often those who claim that there is no god (atheists) are those being considered as unreasonable and even impaired? Why is it then that religious people who pretend to be able to speak to their god, hear him and see him are considered normal? Such behavior should shock us and not generate some form of awe or some sort of admiration and it should be considered a pathological human behavior.

Just what have we encountered in the behavior of those religious people we have considered all through our quest? They all exhibit a belief in something with no basis in reality. They experience, to different degrees, seeing or hearing things that others do not see or hear (hallucinations and/or delusions). Other symptoms may include incoherent speech (called speaking in tongues) and behavior that is inappropriate for the situation (rolling on the floor, exhibiting spasms). They sometimes have difficulty determining what is real and what is not to the point of losing contact with external reality where thought and emotions are impaired even if just momentarily. The consequences of which may be sleep deprivation, social withdrawal and many more.

These people go to church too often because of excessive and irrational anxiety or even obsession over their finances, their marriage, their relationships in general and they expect to find a ready-made recipe for a cure, in fact, they are guaranteed one in the person of a god who loves them more than anyone else and who is all-powerful; "God will heal" is the grand slogan of religion. When one watches how people behave during grand masses in many churches, one wonders just what goes on in the minds of those assembled. It is impossible not to consider some form of epidemic mental disorder and one wonders what type of asylum one has mistakenly wondered into. What is more, when one tries to imagine the incredible sums of money thrown away for the purchase of CDs, DVDs, that promise healing or the purchase of cathedral-like buildings or a new jet for the televangelist/head priest, it is mind boggling. All the while hundreds of thousands of innocent children and adults around the world could use the benefits of medical research this money could go toward, not to mention the water, sanitation and basic life-saving-drugs a simple portion of this money could buy for them. The money wasted to religion is, disgustingly, outrageously inhumane and simply criminally abject and vomitus.

Religion and psychotherapy

We have all known, or known of, persons who have a phobia of witches, devils, evil spirits, black cats, and even, ironically God himself. The term "phobia" refers to a group of anxiety symptoms brought on by certain objects or situations. A phobia is a lasting and unreasonable fear caused by the presence or thought of a specific object or situation that usually poses little or no actual danger. Exposure to the object or situation brings about an immediate reaction, causing the person to endure intense anxiety (nervousness) and the situation can significantly interfere with the person's ability to function. Adults with a specific phobia recognize that the fear is excessive or unreasonable, yet are unable to overcome it; it is pathological.

"A person suffering from a phobia is suffering from a diagnosable illness, a mental health illness that professionals take very seriously. A complete medical and psychiatric evaluation should be conducted by a licensed physician or psychologist. Cognitive-behavioral therapy teaches the persons new skills in order to react differently to the situations which trigger the anxiety or panic attacks. Patients also learn to understand how their thinking patterns contribute to the symptoms and how to change their thinking to reduce or stop these symptoms. No one should have to endure the terror of phobias or the unrelenting anticipatory anxiety that often accompanies them. Phobias can be overcome with proper treatment."[22] (Source: Mental-Health-America).

When this anxiety is so serious that it interferes with work, leads to avoid certain situations or keeps from enjoying life, the person may be suffering from a type of mental disorder; anxiety disorder. Agoraphobia (fear of spiders) is listed in the Diagnostic and Statistical Manual of Mental Disorder Volume 5 (DSM-5) as an anxiety disorder [Dec 20, 2017].

Here are few types of specific phobias, based on the object or situation feared, including:
- Animal phobias: the fear of cats, dogs, snakes, insects, birds, or rats.

- Natural environment phobias: the fear of thunderstorms, Lightening, heights, or even water.
- Bodily-injury phobias: a fear of being injured, of seeing blood or of surgical procedures, and other medical procedures such as blood tests or injections, etc.
- Situational phobias: Involve a fear of specific situations, such as being in a closed-in place, flying, driving, riding in a car or on public transportation, going over bridges or through tunnels, etc.
- Other phobias: fear of heights, a fear of loud noises, and a fear of costumed characters (except perhaps priests).

There is therapy available to those with a fear of heights (Acrophobia), with a fear of spiders (Arachnophobia) and most other phobias. Why then is there no "phobia of the invisible friend" listed and no specific therapy for the fear of this invisible friend (god)?

Though I am not a doctor, I have experienced disturbing behavior on the part of several people I have known over the years of my quest who got up every day and started with the question, "What does god want of me today, what have I done wrong to have earned this scratch on my car or this bump on my head from running into the door?" In these people the guilt-forever-syndrome has attained the level of a neurosis; "I am in eternal sin, therefore I must get used to being in eternal punishment". Any self-respecting psychotherapist, psychoanalyst, and medical doctor will recognize in the short list of above behavioral descriptions the disorders, or potential disorders, running rampant in the religious world. But, this is not a book on clinical cases nor on clinical remedies only a cry for help, a cynical and unabashed look at the seriousness of the religious state of mind from a medical standpoint.

I think that we can all agree that much of this neurosis stems from *"A false belief based on incorrect inference about external reality that is firmly sustained despite what almost everyone else believes and despite what constitutes incontrovertible and obvious proof or evidence to the contrary." (*The belief is one ordinarily accepted by other members of the person's culture or subculture). The preceding definition in italics is that given by the APA and Statistical Manual of Psychology [23] for the term DELUSION. I think that we have sufficiently demonstrated in our quest that the belief (in an invisible friend) is contradicted by so much obvious and convincing evidence that in order to maintain this belief, the believer becomes functionally impaired, and it creates a form of mental suffering for themselves and eventually for others around them. This meets the standards for determining whether a belief is delusional or not. The great Freud thought that religion was delusion and he would agree that religious delusion is out there. It irks me to think that at this very moment, religious institutions are invading the Medical Realm by offering faith-based recovery, "psychiatric care" to hundreds, perhaps thousands of innocent victims; it's like giving victims of sexual abuse back to their abusers for treatment. [23]

Gregg Henriques, Ph.D., author of *A New Unified Theory of Psychology* directs the Combined Clinical and School Psychology Doctoral Program at James Madison University, is a licensed clinical psychologist. He writes; "Although the term *neurotic* has more recently fallen out of favor, it was used by psychiatrists for most of the 20th Century to describe a broad category of conditions that were associated with poor functioning, anxiety and depression, but were clearly differentiated from *psychotic* in that in contrast to individuals in the latter category, neurotics maintained contact with reality and were rarely engaged in highly deviant, socially unacceptable behavior."

This would mean that neurotics don't fall in the psychotic range. He continues, "For a host of reasons, I hope the term makes a comeback, and [... there are ...] various ways the term is still used and how it can be helpful in framing human problems and suffering. The most important thing to distinguish when using the term *neurotic* is to know whether it is referring to personality traits or character adaptations. Personality traits are longstanding patterns of thoughts, feelings, and actions which tend to stabilize in adulthood and remain relatively fixed. There are five broad trait domains, one of which is labeled Neuroticism, and it generally corresponds to the sensitivity of the negative affect system, where a person high in Neuroticism is someone who is a worrier, easily upset, often down or irritable, and demonstrates high emotional reactivity to stress."

I would add that this stress, by the way, can be that of having to renounce to their invisible friend or sometimes simply having to hear someone "insulting" (in their perception) this friend, a reaction that commonly appears in fundamentalists who don't (or can't) understand that one may simply criticize the religion and not the god.

Healing abandoned by Science

As early as the beginning of the 20th Century, Dr. Anton, J. Carlson, a Physiologist at Harvard University delivered an address on "*Science and the Supernatural*" in 1931 where he made his attitude known toward the concept of *Sin*. He states, "The supernatural theories of sin, personified evil, redemption, eternal damnation, etc., when actually believed, have created and are creating much disturbance in man's emotional life, in the way of fear, worry, melancholy, if not outright insanity." That was almost 90 years ago. Why has no one taken heed, why did Medical Science not take measures to intervene in defining and treating religion as a mental illness or at least some of its influences as causal?

Religion likes to throw oil on the flames of fear. All it takes is the fear of damnation or simply the fear of remaining in a state of perceived illness. As I mention in my introduction, god and religion are presented as the ultimate healer of all the ailments one may have. Most of these ailments are psychological; bad marriage, unemployment, addictions, loneliness, and all sorts of "I'm so unhappy" ailments. It always pretends that all it takes to heal is belief in its god which inevitably leads to giving money to a church or a "healer" or "Psycho-vangelist" of the faith.

Alas, too many people are conned by religion into thinking that they have ailments that either don't exist or that can be cured by the false solutions that they are offered; magic books, magic DVDs and magic prayers... placebos of a dangerous kind that result in long term failures. The mendacity of religion should be condemned and its pervasive effect on troubled minds also. In today's bizarre world we see thousands of men and women who seek and need psychological therapy and guidance faced with two solutions. The first is an institution in which a person with no medical background, no medical certification, tells stories derived from a book of fairytales, puts on a show (Televangelists) that allows them to feel cheery, to laugh at themselves, to forget some of their woes and garner false hopes of a final pleasant supernatural, miraculous solution to all of their ailments. These charlatans are not only misrepresenting psychotherapy but are playing dangerously with the minds of these people who need medical help, not hollow solutions, rhetorical liturgy disguised in comedy and simulacra of relief and guidance, all for a price, but that have the potential of doing them great harm in the long run.

At the other end of the spectrum, they have the option of going to see people in lab-coats, in white sterile clinical rooms that make them feel like they are going in for a funeral or a frontal lobotomy, for a solution to what they perceive as an erroneously diagnosed ailment they can never cure from. It is not rocket science to understand that what these people need is medical assistance from a licensed and qualified psychiatrist or psychologist. These people are too ill and too manipulated to see that they are ill, just like hoarders who refuse to admit that they are. They ironically give what little money they may have to charlatans (which include priests and theologians), crystal ball gazers and outright sharks; millions of dollars-worth. Medical science needs to bridge the gap and try to present itself with less drama involved, in a more inviting and understanding manner, but with assurance, guidance and effectiveness. A psychiatrist is a trained medical doctor. He can prescribe medications, and they spend much of their time with patients on medication management as a course of treatment. Psychologists focus extensively on psychotherapy and treating the emotional and mental suffering in patients with behavioral issues. These doctors are certainly losing out on millions of dollars given to these charlatans of televangelism and just plain Churches. They are also losing out on the opportunity to make a difference and truly help these people.

What good is a profession such as psychotherapy, and psychology in general, if it refuses to identify and acknowledge the origins of the disorders it hypothetically is meant to diagnose and treat? The willingness of superstitious people to die for their imaginary, invisible friend is in itself a sign of deep insanity, especially when it involves killing innocent others as well. Medical doctors need to speak up and even get up and find better ways to reach their potential patients. There are TV shows that speak of hoarding problems and of malnutrition for example, with licensed MD's. Leaving things be, is not a good alternative either because these potential patients are being abused and conned out of their money and their mental health. I can't help but feel that these people are being abandoned by medical science because of some unspoken taboo attached to all that is religious; religions that literally sell magic potions and "opioids" to those who need it the least. It isn't without some irony when we compare these lost souls to the lepers that even science rejected as late as the 19th century (G. H. Armauer Hansen in Norway in 1873). How many more Centuries will it take for psychiatric medicine to come to the aid of these people who obviously need it now?

Time wasted to illusions instead of knowledge

Religion has only helped prolong suffering by oppressing medical research, delaying technical advances by burning at the stake the few intelligent souls such as Giordano Bruno, tried and burned for heresy by the Roman Inquisition in 1600, who dared question the skies rendered taboo, among other things, by religious dogmas. If you think that this is just ancient history, think again. In 1981, the Vatican invited a number of experts, including Stephen Hawking, to advise them on cosmology (of all things). The Pope himself (John Paul II) saw each scientific expert individually, after the conference, to tell them that "it was all right to study the evolution of the universe after the big bang, but that they should not inquire into the Big Bang itself because that was the moment of creation and therefore the work of God and the domain of the Church".

Every religion pretends to have the solution to global love, understanding and compassion without realizing that it propagates segregation and inequalities because it can never compromise on its so-called truth. It is not because people believe the world in a specific way, but because they adhere to an institution, an organized clan of believers with an agenda and dogmas, that we will never succeed in ridding ourselves of segregation, and of a plethora of other plagues, through bigotry, superstition and religious terrorism. This is where religion has this despicable agenda of forcing every soul to believe in a specific invisible friend to the point of unbridled warfare, embellished with dismemberments, wholesale genocides, burnings, rapes and other atrocities that good manners do not allow me to list here. Religion does not really care about helping the individual; it is not about good will. This is where religion becomes an intolerant, vindictive, tyrannical power. This is how it has been able to dominate the social and political scene for over 2000 years without ever succeeding in making this place a better world for all men and women.

Yet we respect, we applaud, we adulate and even revere religious figures, both men and women, who know nothing more than any normal individual about the magic man in the sky. I say that many of these people are either lying to themselves, lying to their flock and/or need serious medical treatment. Pursuing a "relationship" as it is called with something that doesn't exist or that we have no access to is not only preposterous but a sign of mental disorder. It should be frowned open and seen as the sign of a Bronze-Age mind; it is an ignominious state of mind unworthy of human kind.

It's not only time to relegate religion to the past but to offer therapy to the masses that need it. So I say to the medical community, "You are missing out on a lot of work and opportunities of the kind of good Hippocrates was talking about. This opens large doors to therapeutic opportunities and new fields of research and to the study of the history of psychotics in religion over the last 2 millennia for example; hallucinations, illusions, ecstasies, delusions and more.

The epitome of all of this is that religion's purpose is death. It awaits impatiently the return of its Christ, Armageddon, the destruction of Earth, and the death of mankind for the "rebirth" of humanity. Meanwhile, humanity awaits impatiently the death of religion for the rebirth of reason and for the next step in the evolution of mankind. Humanity needs to ask itself, as a species, what it wants. Is it is going to be 'God for all and every man for himself' like it has been for the last 4000 years, or is it finally going to apply those wondrous moral principles that scriptures are supposed to be about and that religions have failed to put into application. Moreover, if God does not exist, it's more than time to get our act together and start counting on our mutual compassion, fraternity and wisdom rather than some illusive heaven or 'second coming' to make it happen, because from what Science shows, extinction is forever.

Fairytale land

Even today grown men and women of all walks of life, continue to bow down to grown men in absurd suits depicting an anachronism short of a ridiculous charade or phantasmal parade of dark-age ignorance. Remove their vividly colored habits, their effeminate robes and you will find a man who puts his pants on one leg at a time just like any other man. Society should define religion and religiousness, (as opposed to spirituality and belief), as a neurosis, a syndrome, a paranoia, a delusional pathology or any of a number of other behavioral disorders and treat it as such. Why do the media still parade it as a higher status of intelligence instead of a sign or stage of primitiveness that refuses to evolve?

We can choose to be heartless, mindless, egoistical parasites or we can choose to be compassionate, empathetic, generous, understanding and loving beings. There is no need for religion for us to access Humanism. The degree of our humanism is directly proportional to our degree of intelligence. But, we too often choose to be naïve, superstitious, ignorant, arrogant, gullible and prefer Bronze-Age myths and legends about something invisible, all-merciful, all-intelligent that will show us the way, if only we bow down to the priests that tell us that they know what this invisible, supernatural, and unknowable thing is, when in reality they have no way of communicating with it.

There is much more glory and merit in being human, empathetic, compassionate, etc. simply because, in all logic, it is the right thing to do if we want a better world than there is in torturing one's mind and even that of others by twisting reality to fit an expired scheme that does not work. A scheme that is absurd and that demands that we be hypocrites by believing just to be safe in an invisible something, called God that no one can really understand or really communicate intelligibly with. A concept of a god who loves but who kills for no good reason, a god who is all-intelligent but incapable of sending us a few short manuals on how to be good humans and who sends us instead poems and stories of myths and legends that we torture our minds trying to understand. We have to call out religion for what it really is; a mental disorder-creating and sustaining melanoma that just won't die for lack of therapy.

A rational look at life is frightening at first but very liberating in the long run. We are a part of a fascinating and very real line of evolution. We are a part of the struggle for life. We are predators just like any other animal. But, we are evolved enough to comprehend our place in the cycle of life and death. Our potential for understanding that we are all in this same situation, however frightening, is what makes us Human. Religion might have been useful at one time to help us coalesce, help us become somewhat more civilized, but it is obsolete and has been for centuries. It is time to finally wake up to this reality and to send religion back to the fairytale land that it should have never been allowed to leave.

Appendix

Chapter 1:

[1] Victor Stenger; (January 29, 1935-August 25, 2014) Was an American particle physicist, author and religious skeptic (University of Hawaii) p.4

[2] Daniel Dennett; (born March 28, 1942) is an American philosopher, writer, and cognitive scientist (Tufts University) p4

Chapter 2:

[3] * Theresa Marie "Terri" Schiavo (Died March 31, 2005) was a right-to-die legal case in the United States from 1990 to 2005, a woman in an irreversible persistent vegetative state. Terri's husband and legal guardian argued that she would not have wanted prolonged artificial life support without the prospect of recovery, and elected to remove her feeding tube. The highly publicized and prolonged series of legal challenges presented by her parents ultimately involved state and federal politicians up to the level of President George W. Bush and caused a seven-year delay before Terri's feeding tube was ultimately removed. p8

[4] Study of the Therapeutic Effects of Intercessory Prayer (STEP) in cardiac bypass patients; a multicenter randomized trial of uncertainty and certainty of receiving intercessory prayer; 2005. p12

[5] * https://patch.com/florida/southtampa By David Rice, July 2, 2012 4:02 pm ET & Updated Jul 3, 2012 at 1:51 pm ET. p12

[6] * April 20, 2001: Veronica Bowers and her 7 month old baby Charity were killed by the same bullet in Northeastern Peru by military planes who thought they were drug smugglers. She and her husband Jim Bowers, 37 at the time, from Muskegon, Michigan were Baptist Missionaries. p13

Chapter 4:

[7] *Source: [https://www.jw.org/en/bible-teachings/questions/see-god/ p23

Chapter 6:

[8] Life size Noah's Ark in Kentucky built by Ken Ham; see, arkencounter website. Theme park opened in July 2016. p39

[9] Bill Nye or William Sanford; (November 27, 1955 to present), also known as Bill Nye the Science Guy. American science educator, television presenter, and mechanical engineer. Known for hosting the PBS children's science show (1993–1998), and for being a science educator. p40

[10] Eberhardt Zimmermann, 1777; Specimen Zoologiae Geographicae Quadrupedum p40

[11] The Secular Ark by Janet Browne, 1983 p40

Chapter 7:

[12] Francesco Petrarch (1304-1374 A.D.):
Italian scholar, poet and historian. The first great medieval explorers of History, focused on accuracy. p47

[13] Lorenzo Valla (1407-1457) Italian humanist, pioneer of truth in history convicted of heresy, on eight counts, by the Inquisition and condemned to burn at the stake, after demonstrating that the Apostle's Creed could not have been composed by the twelve Apostles. He was rescued by the King of Italy (Stanford Encyclopedia of Philosophy). p47

[14] Daniel J. Boortin author of The Discoverers, 1985 ISBN# 0-394-72625-1. p47

[15] Bart D. Ehrman; chairs the Department of Religious Studies at the University of North Carolina at Chapel Hill. author of *Misquoting Jesus*. p50

Chapter 9:

[16] David Hume; (born May 7 April 26, 1711, Edinburgh, Scotland — died August 25, 1776, Edinburgh), Scottish philosopher, historian, economist, and essayist known especially for his philosophical empiricism and skepticism. p62

Chapter 10:

[17] See; [https://www.lds.org/topics/prophets?lang=eng] p69

[18] Don Cuppit; (born 22 May 1934 in England) is an English philosopher of religion and scholar of Christian theology, Anglican priest and a professor of The University of Cambridge. p71

Chapter 11:

[19] Karen Armstrong; (British author and commentator) writes in her book, the Case for God (2009), page 308, 174 word quote (Fair Use). p81

[20] Pope Francis; declaration of October 2014; http://www.nowtheendbegins.com/pope-francis-says-genesis-account-creation-true/; Article by Geoffrey Grider p82

Chapter 12:

[21} See, Youtube video with Richard Dawkins; https://www.youtube.com/watch?v=JKGtcVoBhBQ. p87

[22] Source: Mental-Health-America. p90

[23] Article by Lindsay Holmes and Beth Shelburne 09/20/2017 05:46am ET | Updated June 4, 2018; [https://www.huffintonpost.com/entry/finding-mental-health-help-in-faith-based-recoveryus 59c2f462e4b09fd2cbccb9cb] p91

BIBLIOGRAHY & Suggested Readings

(Invisible Friend)

- **Blackburn**, Simon; ***Think***, 1999, ISBN# 0-19-210024-6
- **Boorstin**, Daniel, J.; ***The Seekers***, ISBN# 0-394-40229-4
- **Browne**, Janet; ***The Secular Ark***, 1983, ISBN# 0-300-02460-6
- **Burns**, Edward McNall; ***World Civilizations***, 1995 ISBN# 0393-95517-6
- **Carlson,** Anton J**.**; ***Science and the Supernatural***, in the *Scientific Monthly*, 1931 and reprinted August, 1944
- **Christopher**, John, B.; ***The Islamic Tradition***, 1972, ISBN# 06-041283-6
- **Davies**, Paul; ***God and the New Physics***, 1983, ISBN# 0-671-47688-2
- **Davies**, Paul; ***The Mind of God***, 1992, ISBN# 0-671-68787-5
- **Dawkins**, Richard; ***The God Delusion***, 2006, ISBN# 0-618-680004
- **Ehrman**, Bart D.: ***Misquoting Jesus,*** ISBN# 978-0-06-085951-0
- **Eiseley**, Loren**;** ***Darwin's Century,*** 1961, ISBN# 0-385-08141-3
- **Fairservis**, Walter Jr.; ***The Threshold of Civilization***, SBN# 0-684-14045-4
- **Frankl**, Viktor E.; ***Man's Search for Meaning***, 1959, ISBN# 0-671-66736-X
- **Graham M.**, Lloyd**;** ***Deceptions and myths of the Bible***, 1975, Citadel Press, ISBN# 0-8065-1124-9
- **Hamilton,** Edith; **Mythology: Timeless tales of gods and heroes, 1969, The New American Library Inc.**
- **Heschel**, Abraham, J.; ***Who is Man?*** 1963
- **Hitchens**, Christopher; ***God is not Great***, 2007, ISBN# 978-0-446-69796-5
- **Irvine**, William; ***Apes, Angels and Victorians***, 1955, ISBN# 0-8094-3674-4
- **Johnson**, Luke Timothy; ***The Creed***, 2003, ISBN# 0-385-50247-8
- **Kauffmann**, Walter; ***Existentialism from Dostoevsky to Sartre***, 1975, ISBN# 0-452-00-30-8

- **Le Van Baumer**, Franklin; *Main Currents of Western Thought*, 1978, ISBN# 0-300-02162-3
- **Lombardo,** Stanley; *Homer Iliad,* 1997, ISBN# 0-87220-3530
- **Mencken**, H. L.; *Treatise on the Gods*, 1930, ISBN# 0-8018-5654-X
- **Messadie**, Gerald; *L'Homme qui devint dieu*, 1989, ISBN# 2-221-05597-7
- **Olcott**, Henry, S. ; *The Buddhist Catechism*, 1947, ISBN# 0-8356-0027-0
- **Parrinder**, Geoffrey; *A Dictionary of Non-Christian Religions*, 1971, ISBN# 0-664-20981-
- **Sagan**, Carl; *The Demon Haunted World*, 1996, ISBN# 0-345-40946-9
- **Sagan**, Carl; *Billions and Billions*, 1997, ISBN# 0-679-41160-7
- **Sagan**, Carl; *Contact*, 1985, ISBN# 0-671-43400-4
- **Sagan**, Carl; *Cosmos*, 1980, ISBN# 0-394-50294-9
- **Sagan**, Carl; *Broca's Brain*, 1980, ISBN# 0-394-5
- **Sagan**, Carl; *The Dragons of Eden*, 1977, ISBN# 0-345-28153-5
- **Shapley**, Harlow; *A treasury of Science*, 1943
- **Smith**, Homer, W.; *Man and His Gods*, 1952, ISBN# 0-448-00005-9
- **Taylor**, Alfred E.; *Socrates, the man and his thought*, 1933
- **Teilhard de Chardin**, Pierre; *The Phenomenon of Man*, 1965
- **Warner**, Martin; *Religion and Philosophy*, 1992, ISBN# 0-521-42951-X
- **Young**, Perry Deanne; *God's Bullies*, 1982, ISBN# 0-03-059706-4
- **Zimmermann**, Eberhardt, 1777; *Specimen Zoologiae Geographicae Quadrupedum*

Illustration Credits

All images and illustrations appearing throughout are from the author's collection or own creation.

Also by the Author;

Donc vous avez un ami invisible (French version)

So you have an invisible fear

Donc vous avez une peur invisible

www.ingramcontent.com/pod-product-compliance
Lightning Source LLC
Chambersburg PA
CBHW021441210526
45463CB00002B/601